Minimally Invasive Pediatric Urologic Surgery

Editor

ASEEM R. SHUKLA

UROLOGIC CLINICS OF NORTH AMERICA

www.urologic.theclinics.com

Consulting Editor

SAMIR S. TANEJA

February 2015 • Volume 42 • Number 1

ELSEVIER

1600 John F. Kennedy Boulevard • Suite 1800 • Philadelphia, Pennsylvania, 19103-2899

http://www.theclinics.com

UROLOGIC CLINICS OF NORTH AMERICA Volume 42, Number 1
February 2015 ISSN 0094-0143, ISBN-13: 978-0-323-35453-0

Editor: Kerry Holland
Developmental Editor: Susan Showalter

Urologic Clinics of North America (ISSN 0094-0143) is published quarterly by Elsevier Inc., 360 Park Avenue South, New York, NY 10010-1710. Months of issue are February, May, August, and November. Business and Editorial Offices: 1600 John F. Kennedy Blvd., Suite 1800, Philadelphia, PA 19103-2899. Periodicals postage paid at New York, NY and additional mailing offices. Subscription prices are $355.00 per year (US individuals), $602.00 per year (US institutions), $415.00 per year (Canadian individuals), $752.00 per year (Canadian institutions), $515.00 per year (foreign individuals), and $752.00 per year (foreign institutions). Foreign air speed delivery is included in all *Clinics* subscription prices. All prices are subject to change without notice. **POSTMASTER:** Send address changes to *Urologic Clinics of North America*, Elsevier Health Sciences Division, Subscription Customer Service, 3251 Riverport Lane, Maryland Heights, MO 63043. Customer Service: 1-800-654-2452 (US). From outside the United States, call 1-314-447-8871. Fax: 1-314-447-8029. E-mail: JournalsCustomerServiceusa@elsevier.com (for print support) and JournalsOnlineSupport-usa@elsevier.com (for online support).

Reprints. For copies of 100 or more, of articles in this publication, please contact the Commercial Reprints Department, Elsevier Inc., 360 Park Avenue South, New York, New York 10010-1710. Tel.: 212-633-3874; Fax: 212-633-3820; E-mail: reprints@elsevier.com.

Urologic Clinics of North America is covered in MEDLINE/PubMed (*Index Medicus*), *Excerpta Medica, Current Contents/ Clinical Medicine, Science Citation Index,* and *ISI/BIOMED.*

PROGRAM OBJECTIVE
The goal of *Urologic Clinics of North America* is to keep practicing urologists and urology residents up to date with current clinical practice in urology by providing timely articles reviewing the state of the art in patient care.

TARGET AUDIENCE
Practicing urologists, urology residents and other health care professionals practicing in the discipline of urology.

LEARNING OBJECTIVES
Upon completion of this activity, participants will be able to:
1. Describe the simulation and training as educational methods for pediatric laparoscopists and robotic surgeons.
2. Review laparoscopic orchiopexy, varicocelectomy, nephrectomy, pyelopasty and uretal implantation.
3. Discuss robotic assisted uretal reimplantation, bladder neck repair, appendicovesicostomy and bladder augmentation.

ACCREDITATION
The Elsevier Office of Continuing Medical Education (EOCME) is accredited by the Accreditation Council for Continuing Medical Education (ACCME) to provide continuing medical education for physicians.

The EOCME designates this enduring material for a maximum of 15 *AMA PRA Category 1 Credit*(s)™. Physicians should claim only the credit commensurate with the extent of their participation in the activity.

All other health care professionals requesting continuing education credit for this enduring material will be issued a certificate of participation.

DISCLOSURE OF CONFLICTS OF INTEREST
The EOCME assesses conflict of interest with its instructors, faculty, planners, and other individuals who are in a position to control the content of CME activities. All relevant conflicts of interest that are identified are thoroughly vetted by EOCME for fair balance, scientific objectivity, and patient care recommendations. EOCME is committed to providing its learners with CME activities that promote improvements or quality in healthcare and not a specific proprietary business or a commercial interest.

The planning committee, staff, authors and editors listed below have identified no financial relationships or relationships to products or devices they or their spouse/life partner have with commercial interest related to the content of this CME activity:
Blake B. Anderson, MD; Thane A. Blinman, MD; Paul R. Bowlin, MD; Pasquale Casale, MD; Andrew J. Cohen, MD; Sean T. Corbett, MD; Walid A. Farhat, MD; Ronnie G. Fine, MD; Israel Franco, MD, FACS, FAAP; Patricio C. Gargollo, MD; Mohan S. Gundeti, MB, MCh, FEBU, FRCS (Urol) FEAPU; Kerry Holland; Brynne Hunter; Venkata R. Jayanthi, MD; Chester J. Koh, MD, FACS, FAAP; Indu Kumari; Sandy Lavery; Christopher J. Long, MD; Jill McNair; Rajendra B. Nerli, MBBS, MS, MCh; Joseph J. Pariser, MD; Shane M. Pearce, MD; Mallikarjuna N. Reddy, MS, MCh, DNB, FEBU; Megan S. Schober, MD, Ph.D.; Aseem R. Shukla, MD; Mesrur Selcuk Silay, MD, FEBU; Arun K. Srinivasan, MD; Megan Suermann; Gregory E. Tasian, MD, MSc, MSCE.

The planning committee, staff, authors and editors listed below have identified financial relationships or relationships to products or devices they or their spouse/life partner have with commercial interest related to the content of this CME activity:
Samir S. Taneja, MD is a consultant/advisor for Bayer HealthCare Pharmaceuticals, Eigen Pharma LLC, GTx, Inc., HealthTronics, Inc. and Hitachi, Ltd.

UNAPPROVED/OFF-LABEL USE DISCLOSURE
The EOCME requires CME faculty to disclose to the participants:
1. When products or procedures being discussed are off-label, unlabelled, experimental, and/or investigational (not US Food and Drug Administration [FDA] approved); and
2. Any limitations on the information presented, such as data that are preliminary or that represent ongoing research, interim analyses, and/or unsupported opinions. Faculty may discuss information about pharmaceutical agents that is outside of FDA-approved labelling. This information is intended solely for CME and is not intended to promote off-label use of these medications. If you have any questions, contact the medical affairs department of the manufacturer for the most recent prescribing information.

TO ENROLL
To enroll in the *Urologic Clinics of North America* Continuing Medical Education program, call customer service at 1-800-654-2452 or sign up online at http://www.theclinics.com/home/cme. The CME program is available to subscribers for an additional annual fee of USD $270.

METHOD OF PARTICIPATION
In order to claim credit, participants must complete the following:
1. Complete enrolment as indicated above.
2. Read the activity.
3. Complete the CME Test and Evaluation. Participants must achieve a score of 70% on the test. All CME Tests and Evaluations must be completed online.

CME INQUIRIES/SPECIAL NEEDS
For all CME inquiries or special needs, please contact elsevierCME@elsevier.com.

Contributors

CONSULTING EDITOR

SAMIR S. TANEJA, MD
The James M. Neissa and Janet Riha Neissa
Professor of Urologic Oncology; Professor of
Urology and Radiology; Director, Division of
Urologic Oncology; Co-Director, Smilow
Comprehensive Prostate Cancer Center,
Department of Urology, NYU Langone Medical
Center, New York, New York

EDITOR

ASEEM R. SHUKLA, MD, FAAP
Director, Minimally Invasive Surgery,
Division of Urology, Children's Hospital of
Philadelphia; Associate Professor of Surgery
(Urology), Perelman School of Medicine,
University of Pennsylvania, Philadelphia,
Pennsylvania

AUTHORS

BLAKE B. ANDERSON, MD
Pediatric Urology, Section of Urology,
The University of Chicago Medical Center and
Comer Children's Hospital, Chicago, Illinois

THANE A. BLINMAN, MD
Assistant Professor of Surgery, Division of
General, Thoracic and Fetal Surgery,
Children's Hospital of Philadelphia,
Philadelphia, Pennsylvania

PAUL R. BOWLIN, MD
The Hospital for Sick Children, Toronto,
Ontario, Canada

PASQUALE CASALE, MD
Chief, Department of Urology, Morgan Stanley
Children's Hospital; Professor of Urology,
Columbia University Medical Center,
New York, New York

ANDREW J. COHEN, MD
Pediatric Urology, Section of Urology, The
University of Chicago Medical Center and
Comer Children's Hospital, Chicago, Illinois

SEAN T. CORBETT, MD
University of Virginia Children's Hospital,
University of Virginia, Charlottesville, Virginia

WALID A. FARHAT, MD
The Hospital for Sick Children, Toronto,
Ontario, Canada

RONNIE G. FINE, MD
Cohen Children's Medical Center, Hofstra
North Shore-LIJ School of Medicine,
Long Island, New York

ISRAEL FRANCO, MD, FACS, FAAP
New York Medical College, Valhalla,
New York

PATRICIO C. GARGOLLO, MD
Co-Director, Urology Robotic and Minimally
Invasive Surgery Program; Attending Surgeon,
Division of Pediatric Urology, Department of
Surgery; Associate Professor of Urology,
Baylor College of Medicine; Director, Program
for Complex Urogenital Reconstruction, Texas
Children's Hospital, Houston, Texas

**MOHAN S. GUNDETI, MB, MCh, FEBU,
FRCS (Urol), FEAPU**
Pediatric Urology, Section of Urology,
The University of Chicago Medical Center
and Comer Children's Hospital, Chicago,
Illinois

VENKATA R. JAYANTHI, MD
Chief, Pediatric Urology, Section of Pediatric
Urology, Nationwide Children's Hospital;
Clinical Associate Professor, Department of
Urology, The Ohio State University School of
Medicine, Columbus, Ohio

CHESTER J. KOH, MD, FACS, FAAP
Associate Professor and Pediatric Robotic
Surgery Program Director, Division of Pediatric
Urology, Department of Surgery, Texas
Children's Hospital; Scott Department of
Urology, Baylor College of Medicine,
Houston, Texas

CHRISTOPHER J. LONG, MD
Pediatric Urology Fellow, Division of
Urology, Children's Hospital of Philadelphia,
Perelman School of Medicine, University of
Pennsylvania, Philadelphia, Pennsylvania

RAJENDRA B. NERLI, MS, MCh
Division of Pediatric Urology, Department of
Urology, Director, KLES Kidney Foundation,
KLES Dr Prabhakar Kore Hospital and MRC,
KLES University's JN Medical College,
Belgaum, India

JOSEPH J. PARISER, MD
Pediatric Urology, Section of Urology,
The University of Chicago Medical Center
and Comer Children's Hospital, Chicago,
Illinois

SHANE M. PEARCE, MD
Pediatric Urology, Section of Urology, The
University of Chicago Medical Center and
Comer Children's Hospital, Chicago, Illinois

MALLIKARJUN N. REDDY, MS, MCh
Division of Pediatric Urology, KLES Kidney
Foundation, KLES University's JN Medical
College, Belgaum, India

MEGAN S. SCHOBER, MD, PhD
Pediatric Urology Fellow, Section of Pediatric
Urology, Nationwide Children's Hospital,
Columbus, Ohio

ASEEM R. SHUKLA, MD, FAAP
Director of Minimally Invasive Surgery,
Associate Professor of Urology in Surgery,
Children's Hospital of Philadelphia, Perelman
School of Medicine, University of
Pennsylvania, Philadelphia, Pennsylvania

MESRUR SELCUK SILAY, MD, FEBU
Research Fellow, Division of Pediatric Urology,
Department of Surgery, Texas Children's
Hospital; Scott Department of Urology, Baylor
College of Medicine, Houston, Texas

ARUN K. SRINIVASAN, MD
Assistant Professor of Urology in Surgery,
Division of Urology, Children's Hospital of
Philadelphia, Perelman School of Medicine,
University of Pennsylvania, Philadelphia,
Pennsylvania

GREGORY E. TASIAN, MD, MSc, MSCE
Assistant Professor, Division of Urology,
Department of Surgery, Center for Pediatric
Clinical Effectiveness, Children's Hospital of
Philadelphia, Perelman School of Medicine,
University of Pennsylvania, Philadelphia,
Pennsylvania

MATTHEW D. TIMBERLAKE, MD
University of Virginia Children's Hospital,
University of Virginia, Charlottesville, Virginia

DANA A. WEISS, MD
Assistant Professor of Urology in Surgery,
Perelman School of Medicine, University of
Pennsylvania, Philadelphia, Pennsylvania

Contents

> The increasing incidence of pediatric stone disease has coincided with significant advances in technology and equipment, resulting in drastic improvements in management. Miniaturization of both ureteroscopes and percutaneous nephrolithotomy (PCNL) equipment has facilitated access to the entirety of the urinary tract and has made ureteroscopy a first-line therapy option along with shockwave lithotripsy for kidney and ureteral stones. Advances in PCNL have decreased patient morbidity while preserving stone clearance rates. In this review, the advances in operative approach for ureteroscopy and PCNL in children and its applicability to current surgical management of pediatric stone disease are discussed.

> The role of laparoscopy in the case of nonpalpable cryptorchidism is both diagnostic and therapeutic. Laparoscopic orchiopexy for nonpalpable testes in the pediatric population has become the preferred surgical approach among pediatric urologists over the last 20 years. In contrast, laparoscopic varicocelectomy is considered one of several possible approaches to the treatment of a varicocele in an adolescent; however, it has many challengers and it has not gained universal acceptance as the gold standard. This article reviews the published evidence regarding these surgical techniques.

 Videos of umbilical incision, trocar incision, colon mobilization, transperitoneal nephrectomy, and prone nephrectomy accompany this article

> The indication for use of laparoscopy, in the pediatric population, was initially for diagnostic purposes. As confidence with the technology and utility grew, it began to be applied for therapeutic indications. With equivalent surgical outcomes and decreased morbidity, the usefulness of a laparoscopic approach became more apparent, and today minimally invasive surgery is an indispensable tool in the management of many pediatric urologic conditions. The management of renal pathologies using laparoscopy is now currently the approach of choice for most pediatric renal maladies.

Ureteropelvic junction (UPJ) obstruction is a common anomaly, and presents clinically in all pediatric age groups. The past 3 decades have witnessed an evolution in the surgical correction of UPJ obstruction on several fronts, with open surgical techniques yielding way to endoscopic, laparoscopic, and robotic-assisted approaches. Robotic-assisted surgery has several advantages in complex laparoscopic reconstructive procedures such as pyeloplasty. Comparative studies of laparoscopic and robot-assisted repairs have demonstrated similar success rates. Laparoscopic pyeloplasty is here to stay because of its advantages of safety, efficacy, decreased morbidity, reduced hospital stay, and, perhaps most importantly, cost-effectiveness.

 A video of vesicoscopic ureteral reimpantation accompanies this article

Vesicoscopic ureteral reimplantation is a challenging procedure to learn but does have outcomes equivalent to standard open repair. Children objectively have less pain than after an open cross-trigonal repair. Operative times compare favorably to other forms of minimally invasive surgery.

 Videos of robotic-assisted laparoscopic ureteroureterostomy and robotic-assisted laparoscopic partial nephrectomy accompany this article

The optimal management approach for children with ureterocele and complete pyeloureteral duplication, especially in the setting of high-grade ipsilateral vesicoureteral reflux, remains unclear. Trends in surgical management reflect a shift from single-stage open reconstruction toward conservative management and minimally invasive approaches. This article reviews lower tract approaches (endoscopic ureterocele incision and ipsilateral ureteroureterostomy), and upper tract approaches (ureterocele moiety heminephrectomy) in terms of selected operative techniques, patient selection, published outcomes, postoperative care, and follow-up. Current data support endoscopic puncture as a safe and effective treatment of symptomatic children with single-system intravesical ureteroceles.

Bladder and calyceal diverticula are rare clinical entities in the pediatric population. Most of these diverticula are asymptomatic, incidentally detected, and may not require surgical intervention. However, if surgery is indicated, there are minimally invasive treatment options available that have success rates comparable with those of traditional open surgery. In addition, they offer several advantages including reduced morbidity, decreased hospital length of stay, improved cosmesis, and reduced pain medication requirements. In this review, the minimally invasive surgical techniques in the management of bladder and calyceal diverticula are discussed.

Robotic pyeloplasty is now commonly performed for children with ureteropelvic junction obstruction. Because surgical robotics is a tool that facilitates pyeloplasty and other reconstructive urologic operations, the indications for robotic-assisted laparoscopic pyeloplasty are the same as those for an open pyeloplasty but offer distinct advantages with respect to visualization, range of motion, and ease of laparoscopic suturing. In this review, the authors discuss the operative approach for robotic pyeloplasty in children and the extensions of the basic techniques to challenging clinical scenarios.

The development of the robotic-assisted laparoscopic ureteral reimplantation has tracked a path searching for the optimal method of providing outcomes on par with the gold standard of open intravesical ureteral reimplantation combined with fewer complications and decreased discomfort for the patient. With this in mind, pioneers in pediatric urology minimally invasive surgery have put limits to the test with laparoscopic transvesicoscopic Cohen reimplants and laparoscopic extravesical Lich-Gregoir reimplants and then used the da Vinci platform to fine-tune and bring these skills into the 21st century.

Minimally invasive techniques are rapidly being developed and integrated into urologic surgery. Over the past 5 years, the urologic literature is abound with novel techniques and adaptations to conventional laparoscopy. Pediatric urology is no exception to this trend, and the benefits of minimally invasive surgery may be accentuated in children given the relatively more confined working spaces and also a heightened awareness of cosmesis for the pediatric population. Increasingly, complex pediatric urologic procedures are being performed with robot assistance. The feasibility of nephrectomy, pyeloplasty, ureteral reimplantation, and bladder surgery has been clearly established.

There is growing interest in applying robotic-assisted laparoscopic techniques to complex reconstructive pelvic surgery owing to inherent benefits of precision, tissue handling, and articulating instruments for suturing. This review examines preliminary experiences with robotic-assisted laparoscopic augmentation ileocystoplasty and Mitrofanoff appendicovesicostomy (RALIMA) as either an isolated or combined procedure. These series suggest RALIMA is feasible, with the benefit of early recovery and improved cosmetic results in selected patients. The robotic approach incurs functional outcomes and complication rates similar to those of open techniques. Given the steep learning curve, only surgeons with extensive robotic experience are currently adopting this technique.

Minimally invasive surgery (MIS) has changed pediatric urology and general surgery, offering less morbidity and new surgical options for many procedures. This promise goes unrealized when technical methods lag. Application of MIS in children is uneven after more than 2 decades of application. Principles of versatile and proficient technique may remain unstated and implicit in surgical training, often leaving surgical training an exercise in inference and imitation. This article describes some essential practical principles of precision MIS applied to patients of any size.

UROLOGIC CLINICS OF NORTH AMERICA

Foreword
Minimally Invasive Pediatric Urologic Surgery

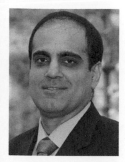

Samir S. Taneja, MD
Consulting Editor

Pediatric Urology is truly a discipline of Urology unto itself. While most of us trained in the basics of the "bread-and-butter" procedures, the practice of Pediatric Urology has evolved to a highly specialized science with techniques and approaches to disease that are often entirely distinct from their Adult Urology counterpart. Nonetheless, an understanding of the contemporary approach to urinary tract disease within the pediatric patient is critically important for every practicing urologist—not just for the ability to counsel patients at time of triage but also to determine if such practices might influence our approach to the adult patient. Much of the innovation in urologic surgical approach, reconstruction, disease management, and perioperative management comes from our pediatric colleagues. Some of the advances are, indeed, specific to the pediatric patient, but many span across the discipline.

Minimally invasive approaches to urologic surgery have revolutionized the surgical management of most common urinary tract disorders. The impact is, perhaps, greatest in the management of pediatric patients. My recollection of pediatric urologic surgery is that of complex procedures performed through small incisions stretched wide open. While such incisions left small scars, the pain children encountered in recovery was certainly considerable. Aside from the commonly thought of impact of minimally invasive procedures on the speed of recovery, the implications on the psychological recovery of the child are broad reaching, ranging from pain and pain medication use to return of appetite to cosmetic outcome. Furthermore, the ability to perform procedures in a minimally invasive pattern, if proven to have less impact on the recovery of the child, may impact on the indications for the surgery itself.

In this issue of *Urologic Clinics*, Dr Aseem Shukla, the Director of Minimally Invasive Surgery at the Children's Hospital of Philadelphia, has created a comprehensive overview of common and emerging minimally invasive procedures in Pediatric Urology. The contributing authors have provided not only a description of the technique but also a discussion of the potential impact of each procedure on the field, and controversies surrounding its use. I am deeply indebted to Dr Shukla and all the contributing authors for this outstanding issue.

Samir S. Taneja, MD
Division of Urologic Oncology
Smilow Comprehensive Prostate Cancer Center
Department of Urology
NYU Langone Medical Center
150 East 32nd Street, Suite 200
New York, NY 10016, USA

E-mail address:
samir.taneja@nyumc.org

http://dx.doi.org/10.1016/j.ucl.2014.10.002

Preface
Minimally Invasive Pediatric Urologic Surgery

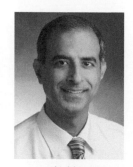

Aseem R. Shukla, MD, FAAP
Editor

While the practice of surgery advanced tremendously due to innovations in anesthesia, analgesia, and antibiotics over the past century, the advent of laparoscopy followed by robotic-assisted laparoscopy is transforming actual surgical approach and technique within the span of little more than the past decade. The surgeon's hands moved first out of the abdomen to working through a trocar, and now are moving from the bedside to the console.

Urologists were early adaptors of robotic-assisted laparoscopy, and pediatric urology similarly led in incorporating the technology into the surgical armamentarium for treating even the smallest infants. And it is in that tradition that this issue of *Urologic Clinics* surveys the journey from the earliest pure laparoscopic procedures to the most advanced reconstruction possible today due to evolutions in technology.

We begin with the procedure that arguably popularized the laparoscopic approach in pediatric urology—the laparoscopic orchiopexy—then posit the continued relevance of pure laparoscopy in the robotic era, before finally surveying contemporary advances in robotic-assisted pediatric urologic surgery. It is my sincere hope that this issue will serve as a necessary guide not only for the novice contemplating a transition to laparoscopy or robotics but also for the seasoned minimally invasive surgeon seeking to enhance skills and augment her practice.

The contributors of the articles herein are not only recognized leaders of minimally invasive surgery globally but also passionate teachers that willingly put forth dedicated efforts to make this issue a reality—and I am indebted to their support. I also express my appreciation to Dr Samir Taneja for conceiving of this endeavor and to Kerry Holland and Susan Showalter at Elsevier for their guidance throughout the process.

To my wife, Suhag, my endless love, and to Parth and Nimai—this is a compilation of where your video gaming skills may one day find their most constructive expression!

With much gratitude,

Aseem R. Shukla, MD, FAAP
Minimally Invasive Surgery
Division of Urology
Children's Hospital of Philadelphia
Perelman School of Medicine
University of Pennsylvania
3rd Floor, Wood Building
34th Street and Civic Center Boulevard
Philadelphia, PA 19104, USA

E-mail address:
shuklaa@email.chop.edu

Urol Clin N Am 42 (2015) xv
http://dx.doi.org/10.1016/j.ucl.2014.10.001
0094-0143/15/$ – see front matter © 2015 Published by Elsevier Inc.

Percutaneous Nephrolithotomy and Ureteroscopy in Children: Evolutions

Christopher J. Long, MD, Arun K. Srinivasan, MD*

KEYWORDS

- Ureteroscopy • Percutaneous nephrolithotomy • Surgical management pediatric stones

KEY POINTS

- The incidence of pediatric nephrolithiasis is increasing.
- Efforts must be made to minimize radiation exposure for both diagnostic and interventional procedures in the pediatric age group.
- Knowledge of the available instrumentation is critical for successful and safe stone removal.
- Miniaturization of equipment and improved optics have facilitated surgical access to all portions of the collecting system and decreased patient morbidity.

INTRODUCTION

The incidence of pediatric stone disease has increased drastically over the past 2 decades, particularly in the adolescent age group.[1–3] This increase in pediatric stone disease has made pediatric urolithiasis an increasingly recognized problem across the world with significant health care cost.[1] In turn, this has coincided with further refinement in the diagnosis, metabolic assessment, and management of the pediatric stone patient. Surgical therapy for pediatric stone disease has undergone significant refinement during that timeframe, decreasing the morbidity of surgical intervention with miniaturization of equipment and drastically improved optics, thereby strengthening the pediatric urologist's armamentarium by significantly improving ureteroscopy (URS) and percutaneous nephrolithotomy (PCNL) for application to children.

EPIDEMIOLOGY

The incidence of stone disease in the pediatric population has been increasing worldwide. Population and institutional studies have revealed a startling increase in stone disease over the past 2 decades, particularly for the adolescent age group (12–17 years of age).[1–3] Review of the Pediatric Health Information System hospitals identified a 10-fold increase from 125 children in 1999 to 1389 in 2008.[4] Identification of systemic risk factors resulting in this increase has identified hypertension, diabetes, salt intake, decreased water intake, and increased/decreased body weight, although the strength of these associations has varied by study.[5,6] Metabolic derangements are common in children and could explain recurrence rates as high as 55% after surgical intervention.[7] Hypocitraturia, hypercalciuria, and oliguria are the most common causes identified in pediatric

---

Division of Urology, The Children's Hospital of Philadelphia, Perelman School of Medicine at the University of Pennsylvania, 3rd Floor, Wood Center, 34th Street and Civic Center Boulevard, Philadelphia, PA 19104, USA
* Corresponding author.
E-mail address: srinivasana3@email.chop.edu

Urol Clin N Am 42 (2015) 1–17
http://dx.doi.org/10.1016/j.ucl.2014.09.002
0094-0143/15/$ – see front matter © 2015 Elsevier Inc. All rights reserved.

24-hour urine assessment.[8,9] Most stones in children are calcium-containing with a much smaller proportion of uric acid compared with adults.[10,11] Contrary to the adult population, girls are slightly more likely to develop stone disease than boys.[1,4,10,12] Boys appear to be more susceptible to developing stones in the first 10 years of life, while this ratio shifts to girls in the second decade.[12] Non-Hispanic whites are more likely to develop stones than Hispanic and black children.[1,4]

IMAGING

The imaging modality of choice in the pediatric population for a suspected stone is either a noncontrast CT scan and/or a renal bladder ultrasound (US). Although US is less sensitive and specific when compared with CT for overall stone recognition, CT scan unfortunately exposes the child to ionizing radiation, thereby increasing their risk of developing cancer.[13,14] Despite these concerns, CT scan utilization is on the rise in the pediatric population, most likely because its sensitivity and specificity for stone diagnosis approach 100%.[15] Although the cancer risk of a single CT scan is low, the fact that stone recurrence is common and can lead to multiple scans over an extended period of time could result in a lifetime of incremental radiation exposure.[13] Comparing the diagnostic effectiveness of combined US and kidneys, ureters, and bladder radiograph (KUB) to CT scan in children presenting with symptomatic stones, the US and KUB resulted in the correct diagnosis 90% of the time.[16] US and KUB were able to diagnose a stone and, if suspicion prompted subsequent CT, a strong argument could be made for them as screening tools. Factors that increase US sensitivity for stone detection include dilation of the ureter and/or pelvis, direct visualization of stones, and the lack of a ureteral jet.[17] In 2012, the American Urological Association released guidelines identifying US as first-line screening tool for urolithiasis with CT scan reserved for situations in which the diagnosis is unclear or if it is necessary for more precise surgical planning.[18] That being said, US poorly identifies ureteral stones and can overestimate stone size, particularly when stones are less than or equal to 5 mm, which can negatively impact surgical planning.[19,20]

WORKUP

The signs and symptoms of stone disease vary in the pediatric population based on age and underlying comorbidities. Older children can present similar to adults with renal colic, abdominal pain, nausea, and vomiting. In younger children, the diagnosis can be much less obvious and can present with hematuria, urinary tract infection (UTI), abdominal pain, nausea, and vomiting. A detailed history for all patients should include identification of any underlying medical conditions and medications, dietary habits including fluid intake, and family history of stone disease.

In general, all children with nephrolithiasis should undergo routine metabolic workup, even first-time stone-formers. This metabolic workup should include a complete metabolic blood panel and a 24-hour urine collection, which should include supersaturation profiles of calcium oxalate, calcium phosphate, and uric acid, which can be elevated even in the setting of normal 24-hour urine values, increasing the risk for stone development.[21] Patients with renal anomalies (ureteropelvic junction [UPJ] obstruction, calyceal diverticulum, vesicoureteral reflux) and those that undergo surgical stone removal warrant further assessment because their risk of recurrence is significantly elevated.[7] Lao and colleagues[7] examined recurrence rates in patients undergoing surgical intervention for stone disease. They found a 5-year overall recurrence rate of 55%, which was significantly more likely to occur for renal stones (93%) than ureteral stones (26%), and those undergoing PCNL (100%) were more likely to recur than those that underwent URS (28%). Hypercalciuria and/or hypocitraturia have been identified in anywhere from 70% to 90% of pediatric patients with urolithiasis and present not only a risk for recurrence but also a target for dietary modification and medical intervention.[7,22,23] Population studies seeking to identify systemic illnesses associated with stone development parallel those in adults have identified hypertension, obesity, and diabetes as systemic illnesses that may increase risks for developing stone disease.[5,24] As insights into the medical aspect of stone disease continue to make gains, this assessment and targeted medical therapy will be able to be incorporated into surgical management to decrease recurrence rates.

Ureteroscopy

Treatment options for pediatric stone disease include shock wave lithotripsy (SWL), URS, PCNL, and open stone removal via an open or a minimally invasive approach. Guidelines published in 2007 identify URS as first-line treatment, along with SWL, in the management of ureteral and renal calculi in the pediatric patient.[25] Before that time, URS was recommended as second-line therapy because of poor instrumentation. Indeed, URS along with SWL has now become the first-line therapy for renal and ureteral stones at many institutions.[26–28]

Technique

The authors' technique is as follows. All patients are administered perioperative intravenous antibiotics and general anesthesia. The patient is then placed in the dorsal lithotomy position. Cystoscopy is performed and intraoperative urine culture is always obtained. The ureteral orifice is cannulated with either a sensor or a guide-wire and an appropriately sized open-ended catheter is inserted to perform a retrograde pyelogram and to determine ureteral diameter and whether it will accommodate the ureteroscope. If it appears as though the ureter is too narrow, a double J stent is placed and a staged URS is performed. If the ureter is of sufficient caliber, a dual lumen catheter is placed and a second wire is inserted. A ureteral access sheath is then placed to facilitate scope passage and stone removal and to decrease ureteral trauma. The authors use the holmium:YAG laser for lithotripsy when appropriate. For intrarenal and proximal ureteral access, they use a 7.5-Fr ureteroscope and for distal stones a 7.5-Fr semirigid ureteroscope. When a ureteral stent is left in place, the authors try to leave a tether when appropriate to facilitate removal; otherwise, it is removed in 1 to 8 weeks endoscopically under general anesthesia. Follow-up consists of US 4 to 8 weeks after URS.

Recent advances

Efforts to decrease radiation exposure in the pediatric population have led to the pursuit of alternative methods to fluoroscopy to facilitate URS. In adult patients, US guidance has successfully facilitated entire procedures, without compromise of operative times, stone-free rates, or complication rates.[29] The authors recognize that although the radiation exposure for a single procedure is low, the recurrent nature of stone disease and the increased susceptibility of the pediatric patient to radiation make minimizing radiation exposure imperative. As such at the authors' institution, they have begun to use US guidance in select routine URS and double J stent insertion procedures in place of fluoroscopy. Alternatively, others have found that intraoperative radiation utilization can be significantly reduced with user education, monitoring, and institution of a radiation safety checklist.[30] Regardless of the method, efforts to minimize or abstain from radiation utilization are imperative in this age group.

Perhaps the biggest advancement facilitating URS in the pediatric patient is equipment miniaturization and advancements in optics. Previously, adult-sized equipment was used in a limited fashion in children. This shift has allowed for retrograde access to the entire collecting system via URS and made it a viable treatment option along with SWL (**Fig. 1**). Semirigid ureteroscopes are now as small as 4.5-Fr and have been used successfully in the pediatric population. A self-dilating 4.5-Fr scope has a tapered tip with a 6.5-Fr body, particularly suited for distal or midureteral stones; this has allowed intubation of smaller-sized ureters without the need for dilation.[31] Authors highlight the atraumatic nature of scope passage, which obviates postoperative stent insertion. Visualization was not impaired as stone free rates after 1 procedure were 97%. The 4.5-Fr Wolf ureteroscope (Wolf, USA) has a 6° lens with a 3.3-Fr working channel that accommodates a 150-μm laser fiber or a 3-Fr basket. An additional advantage of the 4.5-Fr scope was a drastically decreased need for ureteral dilation to remove the stones successfully.[32,33] Further studies have since shown that in children less than 3 years old, the 4.5-Fr ureteroscope offers a distinct advantage in successful stone removal

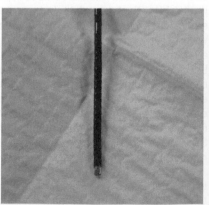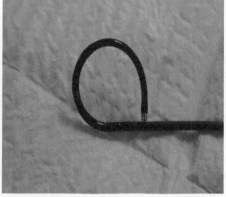

Fig. 1. A 7.5-Fr flexible ureteroscope in unflexed and flexed position.

and complication rates when compared with the 7.5-Fr ureteroscope.[33] One group found no difference in outcomes or complication rates in children undergoing rigid (8-Fr) or semirigid (6.9-Fr) URS.[34]

Active dilation Although advancements in instrument miniaturization have made URS feasible in small children, the ureter does not always accommodate even the smallest of equipment now available. In such cases, options include active or passive ureteral dilation of the ureter and ureteral orifice. Active dilation includes passage of coaxial dilators[26] or dilation with a balloon dilator.[35] Indications for active dilation include a ureter that was not prestented or when difficulty is encountered with scope insertion. The benefit of coaxial dilators versus balloon dilation is the tactile feedback that provides assessment of the ureteral lumen, the determining factor to proceed with ureteral dilation versus stent insertion for passive dilation.[36] Long-term sequelae of active dilation in the pediatric population are unknown at this time and, because most follow-up consists of renal bladder US to look for hydronephrosis, strictures in the absence of significant dilation can be missed.

Passive dilation Passive dilation, on the other hand, involves insertion of a double J stent, and after 1 to 2 weeks the patient's ureter is sufficiently dilated to facilitate scope passage and stone removal. In theory, this approach is less traumatic to the ureter, although a direct comparison in the literature is lacking. One drawback to this approach is that the child is exposed to a second anesthetic to complete the stone removal, and possibly a third if a stent is left without a tether and endoscopic removal is required. Attempts to preoperatively identify patient characteristics, such as height, weight, and body mass index, and correlate them to the ability to perform URS without pre-stenting were inconclusive. The authors were able to use coaxial dilators to successfully perform URS in 13 of 30 (60%) patients, although the remainder required stent placement for passive dilation.[36] The decision to prestent or to dilate is left to the surgeon's discretion and is determined by the ease of catheter, scope, and access sheath passage. It is prudent not to hesitate to place a stent for passive dilation if resistance is encountered. At the authors' institution, they place a stent for when a ureter does not readily accommodate scope passage and rarely pursue active dilation.

Age itself is not a limiting factor for performing successful URS. Mokhless and colleagues[37] published their experience with 21 children with ages ranging from 8 months to 6 years. None of the patients required ureteral dilation, and they were able to navigate the ureter with either a 6.9-Fr rigid miniscope or a 9.5-Fr rigid ureteroscope. They were unable to access the ureter in 1 patient and were able to completely remove the stone burden in 18 of 21 of their cohort. Only 3 of 21 patients required stenting after URS,[37] suggesting that with the appropriate equipment URS remains an option for all age groups.

Ureteral access sheath Ureteral access sheaths facilitate URS by reducing the trauma of repeat scope insertion across the UVJ and distal ureter for stone removal, decreasing intrarenal pressures, and facilitating visualization. These benefits of the ureteral access sheath for adult URS have been proven to carry over in the pediatric population, and in general, they are well tolerated by the smaller-sized ureter, albeit at times only after dilation.[38] Caution must be taken, however, because passage of a ureteral access sheath has been shown to transiently compromise ureteral blood flow, although these changes were not persistent 72 hours after insertion.[39] Complications related to ureteral access sheath center around ureteral perforation and occurred in 6 of 40 cases in a report by Wang et al.[40] Despite a 10% rate of ureteral perforation, the rates of postoperative hydronephrosis did not differ in the sheath group versus the nonsheath group, although definitive excretory studies to rule out ureteral strictures were not performed.[40] In adult patients, ureteral access sheath has resulted in ureteral injury rates as high as 46%, although prestenting the ureter significantly decreased these rates.[41]

Postoperative stenting Postoperative stenting is another practice that is left to the surgeon's discretion. Trials in adult patients have revealed that uncomplicated URS can be safely performed without postoperative stent placement.[42,43] No such randomized trials have been performed in pediatric patients to date but reports in which stents were not left indicate that it was done so without any complications.[26] The decision to leave a stent is based on the duration of the procedure, the degree of ureteral trauma, and the amount of ureteral edema. Stent options include an open-ended catheter that is removed before hospital discharge, an internal double J stent with an externalized tether that can be removed by the family in 3 to 7 days, or an internalized double J stent that is removed under general anesthesia in 1 to 8 weeks.

Options for lithotripsy include ultrasonic, electrohydraulic, laser, and pneumatic lithotripters via URS. The holmium:YAG laser has been directly compared with the pneumatic lithotripter and has resulted in shorter operative times, improved stone-free rates, decreased complications, and decreased stone migration.[44] Many reports have found that the pneumatic device is prone to pushing stones into the proximal ureter, which prolongs operative times, a major disadvantage to its use.[44,45] The holmium:YAG laser is the preferred option for lithotripsy at the authors' institution. All efforts should be made to remove all residual stone fragments regardless of size because in children they are prone to becoming symptomatic with hematuria and/or pain, have a high likelihood of size progression, and have a low likelihood of spontaneous passage.[46]

Complication rates in pediatric URS can be grouped into infection, bleeding, and trauma.[25] Review of the published literature reveals complication rates ranging from 0% to 15% (Table 1).[26,27,31,32,35,37,38,47–58] Infection is encountered most commonly in the form of transient fever, UTI, urosepsis, and/or pyelonephritis. Transient hematuria is the second most commonly encountered entity and rarely requires secondary intervention. Trauma to the small and delicate pediatric anatomy is an obvious concern. Reported rates of ureteral stricture range from 0-2%, although the true incidence of ureteral stricture formation is likely underestimated by the fact that follow up typically consists of renal bladder ultrasound. The true incidence of ureteral stricture formation is unknown because follow-up typically consists of renal bladder US, factors that can underestimate assessment of ureteral stricture formation. Ureteral perforation treated with double J stent insertion is a more common occurrence than ureteral stricture development requiring surgical repair.

A urine culture is recommended for all patients undergoing upper tract manipulation with URS. Antibiotic prophylaxis is recommended before upper tract manipulation. Postoperative antibiotic therapy is controversial. A common theme in pediatric urology is daily antibiotic prophylaxis, but controversy exists regarding the efficacy of this practice as one set of authors found equal UTI risk whether prophylaxis was administered.[59] In the authors' institution, if intraoperative urine culture is negative, then antibiotic prophylaxis is discontinued regardless of stent status unless the patient initially presented with an obstructed, infected stone.

PERCUTANEOUS NEPHROLITHOTOMY

PCNL is more invasive than both SWL and URS, but its safety and efficacy have been well established in the adult literature. Its application in children has evolved and is now a safe and effective option for stone removal. Indications for pursuing treatment via PCNL include large upper tract stone burden (>1.5 cm), lower pole stones greater than 1 cm, concurrent anatomic abnormalities (UPJ obstruction, a duplicated system, urinary diversion), or patients with known cystine or struvite stones.

Technique

The authors' technique is as follows. In general, a PCNL is performed in the prone position. A preoperative CT is obtained to assess the anatomy, and a urine culture is obtained and treated to establish sterility. Access is obtained either by the surgeon or in conjunction with an interventional radiologist. The authors perform a single puncture technique, at times augmented with preoperative ureteral catheter insertion (for contrast or air instillation into the renal pelvis) or under direct vision via a flexible ureteroscope. Once access is obtained, the authors preferentially balloon dilate the tract versus Amplanz renal coaxial dilators. The authors typically use a rigid nephroscope (18 to 24 Fr) or a flexible nephroscope (15-Fr) (Fig. 2). Options for lithotripsy include pneumatic or ultrasonic devices or the holmium:YAG laser. Options for postoperative collecting system drainage include no tube, a nephrostomy tube, an internal double J stent, and a percutaneous nephroureteral catheter. The author's stent size and type preference is dependent upon the age and size of the patient.

Safety

Initial concerns for application of PCNL in children centered on utilization of adult-sized instruments in the pediatric patients and the effects of radiation exposure. The first report of adult instrument use in 7 children aged 5 to 14 years of age resulted in a 100% stone-free rate and no complications.[60] Concerns for renal damage using larger instruments in the relatively smaller pediatric kidney were alleviated with several reports looking at renal scarring in response to intervention. In a pig model, comparison of renal scarring relative to renal parenchyma for a 30-Fr sheath versus an 11-Fr sheath revealed no difference in degree of renal damage as determined by microscopic assessment, suggesting that larger tracts do not result in increased renal unit loss.[61] In a similar porcine model, assessment of renal trauma secondary to tract dilation technique with balloon dilation versus Amplanz sequential dilators revealed no difference in residual scar at 6 weeks after dilation.[62] Samad and colleagues[63] performed follow-up dimercaptosuccinic acid scans after

Table 1
Outcomes and complications in pediatric ureteroscopy

Author	No. Patients/ No. Procedures	Pt. Age, y (mean)	Scope Type	Stone Location (%)	Stone Size, mm (mean)	Stone Free Rate/ Adjunct	Staged/ Preop Stent	Ureteral orifice Dilation	Postoperative Stent: No. (%)	Adjunct Procedures	Complications
al Busaidy et al,[50] 1997	43/50 8.5/9.5/ 11.5 R	0.5–12 (6.2)	8.5 F/9.5/ 11.5 R	100 U	4–22 12.6	84/94	None	12 coaxial 5 balloon	Not provided	Open 3	Fever (12), hematuria (10), stent colic (ureteral perforation with stricture, 1 pt)
Bassiri et al,[48] 2002	66	2–15 (9)	8, 8.5, 9, 11.5 F	100 U	5–15 (8)	88	None	25 balloon	100 (ureteral cath)	8; SWL 4, URS 1, open 3	renal colic (1.5), gross hematuria (17), pyelonephritis (4.5)
Schuster et al,[35] 2002	25/27	0.25–14 (9)	11-Fr R 6.9-Fr F 8-Fr R	7 R 93 U	2–12 (6)	92/100	4 (15)	15 balloon	19 (70)	2 URS	Pyelonephritis (1 pt), stent migration (1 pt)
Satar et al,[51] 2004	33/35	0.8–15 (7.4)	6.9-10-Fr R	100 U	3–10 (5.3)	94	Not reported	11 balloon	12 (34)	1 SWL	Stone migration (1 pt), failed stone removal (1 pt)
Hubert & Palmer,[52] 2005	26/28	7.3–14.1 (10.3)	4.5-8-Fr F, SR	Not reported	Not reported	100	28 (100)	None	None reported	None reported	None reported
Raza et al,[49] 2005	35/52	0.9–15 (5.9)	6.8 Fr, SR	100 U	3–20	72–100	6 (12)	2 coaxial	7 Ureteral cath 4 JJ stent	10 URS	Ureteral perforation (3.8), ureteral stricture (1.9), urinary retention (1.9), transient fever (10)
Minevich et al,[47] 2005	58/65	1–12 (7.5)	6.9 F SR, 7-Fr F	10 P 90 U	Not provided	98	None	20 coaxial 3 balloon	55 (85)	1 SWL	Ureteral stricture (1 pt)
Singh et al,[38] 2006	18	4–13 (9.3)	7.4-Fr F	17 R 83 U	2–14	100	18 (100)	18 sheath	18 (100)	None reported	None reported
Nerli et al,[53] 2011	80/88	6–12 (9.5)	np,F	70 U 30 R	7–16 (10)	90./97.5	25 (31)	Metal tip dilators	Not reported	8; URS 6, SWL 2	Intraop bleeding (7.5), Postoperative bleeding (10), fever (5)

Mokhless et al,[37] 2012	21	0.7–6 (4.7)	7 Fr, 9.5 F	100 U	0.4–13 (6)	90.7	None	None	3 (14)	2 URS	Ureteral perforation (5), stone migration (5), pyelonephritis (5)
Smaldone et al,[26] 2007	100/115	Mean 13.2	6.9 F, F / 7.5 F, SR	94 U / 6 R	Mean 8.3	91	54	70 coaxial / 24 sheath	(76)	7 URS	Ureteral perforation (5), ureteral stricture (1)
Kim et al,[27] 2008	167/170 [54]	0.25–18 (5.1)	8-Fr F	60 P / 40 U	3–24 (6.12)	100 (≤10 mm) / 97 (>10 mm)	95 (57)	None	100	3 URS	None reported
Tanaka et al,[54] 2008	50/52	1.2–13.6 (7.9)	7.5-Fr F	100 R	1–16 (8)	50/9258	17 (33)	18 active / 25 sheath	51 (98)	18; URS 14, PCNL/SWL 4	None reported
Dave et al,[55] 2008	19/28	2–16 (6.9)	7.5-Fr SR	100 R	Mean 17	Pelvis 75 / Polar 100 / Staghorn 14	N/A	8 sheath	N/A	PCNL 1, URS 3, open 2	Ureteral perforation (1 pt), urinoma (1 pt)
Herndon et al,[32] 2006	29/34	2.5–17.5 (11)	4.5-Fr SR / 6.5-Fr SR	100 U	Not reported	96	4 (12)	None	6 (17.6)	1 URS	Ureteral perforation (2 pt)
Uygun et al,[111] 2012	100	0.9–16 (6)	7.5-Fr F / 6.4-Fr SR / 4.5-Fr SR	52 U / 48 R	4–30 (12.8)	81.3 kidney / 100 ureter	44 (44)	44 balloon	61 (61)	9 SWL	Ureteral perforation (2 pts)
Dogan et al,[56] 2011	642/670	0.3–17 (7.4)	4-10-Fr SR	100 U	Mean 8.9	90	207 (30.9)	93 balloon / 113 irrigation pump	61.7 / JJ 74.8 / Ureteral catheter 25.2		Stone migration (1.1), hematuria (1 pt), mucosal laceration (1 pt), ureteral perforation (5 pts), conversion to open (3 pts), pain (2 pts), febrile UTI (20 pts), urinary retention (1 pt), urethral stone (1 pt), UVJ obstruction (4 pts)

(continued on next page)

Table 1
(continued)

Author	No. Patients/ No. Procedures	Pt. Age, y (mean)	Scope Type	Stone Location (%)	Stone Size, mm (mean)	Stone Free Rate/ Adjunct	Staged/ Preop Stent	Ureteral orifice Dilation	Postoperative Stent: No. (%)	Adjunct Procedures	Complications
Yucel et al,[112] 2011	48/54	0.8–18 (7.6)	7.5-Fr SR	100 U	4–20 (6.6)	84.3	2 (4)	4 balloon	31 (61)	4; 3 SWL, 1 URS	Ureteral perforation (1 pt), stone migration (6)
Tiryaki et al,[57] 2013	32/54	0.6–17 (5.9)	4.5-Fr R 7.5-Fr R 7.5-Fr F	100 U	4–18 (8.8)	57/93	8 (19.5)	3 sheath	29 (71)	15; URS	Extravasation (7.3), ureterovesical junction injury (1 pt), nausea/ vomiting (1 pt)
Erkurt et al,[58] 2014	65	0.5–7 (4.3)	7.5-Fr F	100 R	7–30 (26)	83/92	17 (7.7)	40 sheath	N/A	6; URS	Hematuria (9), UTI (15), ureteral injury (3)
Kocaoglu & Ozkan,[31] 2014	36	1–13 (5.3)	4.5-Fr SR	100 U 14 P 14 M 72 D	4–18 (8.4)	97.4/100	None	None	34	1 SWL	Mild hematuria (8), febrile UTI (1 pt), stone migration (1 pt)

Abbreviations: D, distal ureter; F, flexible ureteroscopy; M, middle; np, not provided; P, proximal; R, rigid ureteroscopy; SR, semirigid ureteroscopy; SWL, shock wave lithotripsy; U, ureter URS, ureteroscopy.

Data from Refs. 26,27,31,32,35,37,38,47–58,111,112

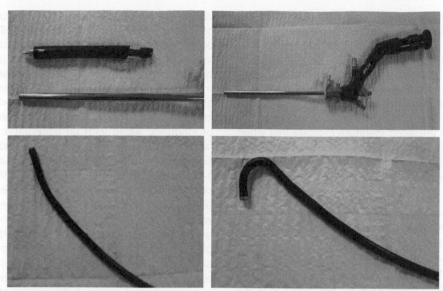

Fig. 2. An 18-Fr pediatric rigid nephroscope, used in the authors' PCNL procedures. The working channel accommodates available lithotriptors, including the laser fiber, Cyberwand, and Lithoclast.

PCNL to look for renal unit loss. They identified 10 of 60 (17%) of renal units with a defect; only 3 (5%) of which were in the site of the working tract and therefore potentially attributed to the procedure. Unfortunately, one limitation to their study was a lack of preoperative renal scans in these patients, making it unclear whether these defects were present preoperatively. Other studies have shown similar preservation of renal function and a lack of scarring in children after PCNL.[64]

Imaging

Before PCNL, preoperative imaging should consist of a helical noncontrast CT. A helical noncontrast CT provides the most accurate assessment of stone burden, identification of any anatomic anomalies that may complicate the procedure and access, and identification of the appropriate calyx for operative approach. Stone scoring systems in adult patients have correlated stone complexity, anatomic considerations, and degree of stone burden as determined by CT scan to operative success and complications.[65,66] Although not validated in children, one could easily see the applicability of a standardized preoperative risk assessment of stone burden that correlates with surgical outcomes. CT scan has been proven superior to other imaging modalities in identifying stone burden and guiding preoperative planning, although as mentioned earlier, efforts must be made to limit exposure to ionizing radiation.[17] Residual stone burden evaluation after PCNL requires a balance between sensitivity of diagnosis and minimizing radiation exposure in the pediatric patient. Radiopaque stones can be evaluated with KUB, which should provide sufficient information regarding stone clearance status, although doing so will underestimate the stone burden, missing up to 45.5% of clinically significant stone fragments (4 mm or greater in diameter).[67] Alternative options for postoperative assessment of stone-free status include CT and US.

Access

Access to the collecting system is a key component to successful stone treatment. Puncture techniques include a US or fluoroscopic-guided approach and can be performed by either a radiologist or the urologist. Single-stick technique is intended to access the collecting system with one puncture to perform PCNL.[68] The 2-stick technique begins with needle insertion to opacify the collecting system to facilitate a second puncture into the desired calyx location.[68] Analysis of urologist-obtained access versus radiologist-obtained access reveals improved stone clearance rates and decreased complications when performed by the urologist.[69–71] The authors propose that the unique understanding of the calyceal anatomy and equipment limitations in conjunction with stone therapy options results in obtaining access more suitable to the full treatment plan. Despite these benefits, most urologists are either deferring access to or performing it in conjunction with a radiologist.[72]

Supracostal access is occasionally required because of anatomic or stone complexity. In particular, large upper pole stones, proximal ureteral stones, concomitant UPJ obstruction, or stones in calyceal diverticulum may need to be accessed via the supracostal approach. This approach increases the risk for lung and pleural injury with resultant hydrothorax or pneumothorax.[73] In addition, there is an increased risk of bleeding, possibly because of the proximity to the intercostal nerve and vessels to the tract site.[74] Reports in the pediatric literature indicate that when necessary this approach can be used with an understanding of the risk of increased complications compared with lower pole access.[75–77]

Drainage

Tubeless PCNL is well established in adults and has been successfully applied to the pediatric population as well.[78,79] Patient selection is key to success and can be applied in all patient ages, even infants.[79] Indications for tubeless PCNL are largely dependent on intraoperative factors, including the degree of dilation, the amount of bleeding encountered, the amount of trauma, the presence of struvite or infectious stones, and collecting system perforation.

The rate of preoperative positive urine culture is less in pediatric patients when compared with adults (15.4%), but at 6% is still significant enough and the consequences of a positive urine culture severe enough that they should be obtained in all patients before instrumentation, particularly the neurogenic bladder population.[76] All patients should also receive perioperative antibiotic prophylaxis.

Technologic Advances

Currently, technology used in adult patients is worth discussing because they often are applied in the pediatric population once efficacy is established. A micro-optic needle scope can be passed via the access needle for direct visual confirmation of access into the collecting system.[80] This micro-optic needle scope has the potential to decrease radiation exposure to the patient and could decrease the number of needle insertions into the kidney. Multiple-access PCNL has become an established option in adults. Its benefits include increased stone clearance and decreased adjunct procedures, albeit with an acceptable morbidity rate.[81] Rate of blood transfusion did increase compared with that in the adult literature to 46 of 149 (30.8%), but stone-free rates and the number of follow-up procedures were decreased. In addition, a Y-puncture technique can be performed in which a single skin puncture site can be used, but the needle is manipulated intracorporeally to pierce the kidney in another calyx to improve stone access.[82] Multiple-access PCNL should be reserved for cases in which complex anatomy or large stone burdens prevent complete stone clearance with a single access. At the authors' institution, they have used multiple-access sites, particularly for large, complex staghorn calculi in the spina bifida patient.

The miniperc further advanced the minimally invasive nature of PCNL.[83] The miniperc has been defined as PCNL performed via a tract of 20-Fr or less and has been further refined with the development of the "micro" and "ultramini" perc.[84] These designations refer to increasingly smaller instrumentation now being used to perform PCNL. These approaches have the advantage of less dilation, a smaller skin incision, and decreased pain for the patient. Tract size has been directly correlated with procedural bleeding and postoperative pain scores.[85] Renal trauma is decreased due to less dilation and torque on the kidney with smaller instruments, which may result in less kidney trauma and allow for routine tubeless PCNL, even in infants.[79] Several

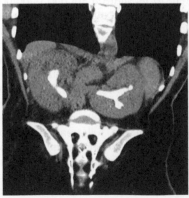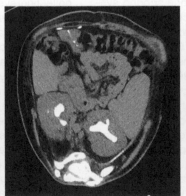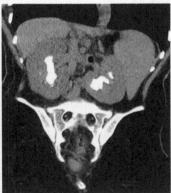

Fig. 3. Bilateral staghorn calculi in a 17-year-old male patient with spina bifida and severe scoliosis. Stone clearance was successful after multiple procedures and access tracts.

Table 2
Percutaneous nephrolithotomy outcomes and complications

Series	No. Patients/ Renal Units	Pt. Age, y (mean)	Stone Size: mm² (mean)	Stone-Free Rate (%) Single Session/ Final	Residual Stones; Adjuvant Therapy	Complications
Mor et al,[91] 1997	22/25	3–16	N/A	68	8; SWL 7, PCNL 3	None long term
Badawy et al,[92] 1999	60/60	3–13	8–37	83.3/90	8; SWL 2, PCNL 4, open 3	Fever (8), transfusion (17), colon injury (2), urine extravasation (3), open conversion (5)
Al-Shammari et al,[93] 1999	8/9	4–11	8–40 (17.4)	87.5	2; SWL 1, anatrophic nephrolithotomy 1	Hypothermia (22)
Zeren et al,[94] 2002	55/62	0.8–14 (7.9)	25–2075 (283)	86.9/96.7	2; open 1, SWL 1	Fever (30), bleeding (23.9), open conversion (2), retained foreign body (2)
Rizvi et al,[95] 2003	62/62	4–14	25–50 (4.7)	68/95	20; SWL 17, open 3	Fever (47), hematuria (21), urine extravasation (6), open conversion (5), hydrothorax (2)
Desai et al,[96] 2004	116/128	6 mo–0.5	110–989 (338)	96.4	6; SWL 3, lost to follow-up 2, spontaneous 1	Infection (5.5), persistent urine leak (2), transfusion (6)
Salah et al,[97] 2004	135/138	8 mo–0.67	124–624 (507)	98.5	1; PCNL	Persistent urine leak (8), transfusion (0.7), fluid collection (0.7)
Raza et al,[98] 2005	37/43	1–15 (6.4)	80–155	79	5; PCNL	Fever (7), pain (7), urine retention (2), renal pelvis tear (7), abscess (2), urine leak, ureteral stricture (2), contrast in inferior vena cava (2), hypothermia (2)
Samad et al,[109] 2006	169/188	0.92–16	33–103	47–90	67; SWL	Fever (44), bleeding (3.7), hyponatremia (5), hypokalemia (4.7)
Shokeir et al,[99] 2006	75/82	0.6–14 (6.6)	12–20	95/100	11; PCNL 7, SWL 4	Fever (2), bleeding (1), pelvis perforation (1)
Bilen et al,[100] 2007	46/53	2–13	26–1582	87–90	4; PCNL 1, SWL 3	Blood transfusion (15), fever (9), urosepsis (6.5), pelvis perforation (6.5), hydrothorax (2)
Roth et al,[101] 2009	24/30	0.6–17.5 (9.6)	25.3	47/97	20; PCNL (2nd look) 16, PCNL 3, SWL 1	Hydrothorax (7), hematuria (3)
Nouralizadeh et al,[102] 2009	20/24	0.5–5 (3.1)	20–46 (33)	79/92	4; PCNL 2, SWL 2	Fever (15), bleeding (5), perforation (5), urine leak (1)

(continued on next page)

Table 2
(continued)

Series	No. Patients/ Renal Units	Pt. Age, y (mean)	Stone Size: mm² (mean)	Stone-Free Rate (%) Single Session/ Final	Residual Stones; Adjuvant Therapy	Complications
Unsal et al,[103] 2010	44/45	0.7–18	14–65	81–83/91–94	Rates not reported; SWL, URS	Bleeding (20), fever (11), pleural effusion (2), UTI (7), transfusion (7), urine leak (5)
Veeratterapillay et al,[104] 2012	31/32	2.8–17.9 (10.8)	5–40 (19)	84/91	5; PCNL 3, SWL 2	Fever (12.5)
Etemadian et al,[110] 2012	38/45	1–13 (8.4)	Mean 29	67	Not reported	Fever (16), transfusion (2), hyponatremia (2)
Bhageria et al,[105] 2013	95/102	3–17 (12)	NA	83/94	18; PCNL 15, 1 URS, SWL 2	Fever (16), sepsis (2), hydrothorax (3), perinephric collection (2), transfusion (9)
Yan et al,[106] 2012	20/27	1.1–5.6 (3.5)	9–28 (18.5)	85.2/92.6	2; SWL	Bleeding (11)
Zeng et al,[87] 2013	331/331	0.7–14 (7.8)	13–36 (2.3)	80/95	54; PCNL 13, URS 11, SWL 27, combined 3	Pain (7), fever (7), infection (4), transfusion (3), pleural injury (0.6), abscess (0.3)
Wah et al,[107] 2013	23/23	1.6–14.6 (4.76)	15–623.44	83.6/90.5	2; PCNL	Hydrothorax (4), infection (13)
Onal et al,[73] 2014	1157/1205	0.33–17 (8.8)	12–212 (4.1)	81.6	4.4% PCNL	Fever (12), pain (1.7), gross hematuria (1), intraoperative transfusion (8), pleural injury (1), hepatic flexure injury (1 pt). pelvis laceration (0.4), urinary extravasation (0.2), febrile UTI (1.6), postoperative transfusion (2.2), hydrothorax (0.3), ureteral stricture (0.2), renal abscess (1 pt), bowel injury (2 pts)
Goyal et al,[108] 2014	153/158	2–17 (10)	150–2400 (377)	85/94	23; PCNL 10, SWL 13	Fever without antibiotics (5), transient urine leak (7.6), hydrothorax (2.5), transient increase in renal function (1.3), transient hematuria (8.2), blood transfusion (7.6), fever with antibiotics (7.6), UTI (0.6), nephrostomy site cellulitis (1.3), hyposaturation on ward (1.3), pneumothorax (1.3), electrolyte anomalies (0.6), UPJ disruption (0.6), bleeding causing procedure termination (2.5), postoperative (0.6)

Data from Refs.[91–110]

reports have indicated a significant decrease in hemoglobin when adult-sized instruments were used in the pediatric population when compared with smaller instrumentation.[85,86] The miniperc system has proven to be a feasible option in select pediatric patients with rates of stone clearance and complications approaching that reported in the adult literature.[87] The microperc consists of a 4.85-Fr single system that contains an "all-seeing" needle that allows for visual confirmation of collecting system during access and provides a working channel for lithotripsy through a very small access sheath.[88] To date, its use is in its infancy because optics are limited compared with the miniperc, and longer operative times have been noted.[88]

Positioning and Anatomic Considerations

Alternative options for patient positioning for PCNL are similar for children as for adults. The traditional prone position is used to decrease bowel complications by dropping the peritoneal contents ventrally away from the access point. There are limits to safe positioning, particularly in obese or contracted patients, such as those with spina bifida. In adults, supine PCNL has been shown to be safe in carefully selected adult patients, with no increase in complication rates, yet was found to have significantly shorter operative times.[89] Some have reported success with supine PCNL in the pediatric patient, although this certainly needs to be done selectively based on anatomic considerations.[76]

Patients with altered anatomy, such as spina bifida patients, caudal regression syndrome, or those with scoliosis, present a particular challenge for stone management (Fig. 3). Although the adult literature has shown that PCNL has successfully been performed in spinal anomalies with minimal complications,[90] this patient population is also of concern for the pediatric urologist. The authors have successfully treated severely contracted patients with staghorn calculi and prefer upper tract access in patients with a previous urinary diversion. A great deal of caution must be undertaken with patient positioning and padding and a CT scan should be performed for obtaining access to the collecting system.

Outcomes and Complications

PCNL is a highly effective intervention when indicated. First-stage stone-free rates range from 47% to 100% and this increases to 90% to 100% when combined with adjunct therapy such as URS, SWL, or second-look PCNL. The degree of stone burden treated must be taken into consideration, which is substantially more compared with that treated by URS or SWL.

As for URS, PCNL complications can be divided into infectious, bleeding, and traumatic causes. Complication rates range from 0% to 30% across the published literature (Table 2).[63,73,87,91–108] Transient fever is the most common complication after PCNL, but urosepsis, pyelonephritis, and febrile UTI are also reported. Bleeding is more common in PCNL compared with alterative endoscopic stone therapies and the rate of transfusion ranges from 0% to 17%. Indications for transfusion vary widely across different reports and no consensus for doing so exists. Issues related to access include bowel, pleural and lung, and vascular injury.

SUMMARY

The increasing incidence of pediatric stone disease has coincided with advances in surgical therapy and has led to improvements in stone diagnosis and reduced radiation exposure. Advances in equipment for both URS and PCNL have decreased the size of the instrumentation and reduced the morbidity of stone removal while simultaneously improving stone removal rates.

REFERENCES

1. Sas DJ, Hulsey TC, Shatat IF, et al. Increasing incidence of kidney stones in children evaluated in the emergency department. J Pediatr 2010; 157(1):132–7.
2. VanDervoort K, Wiesen J, Frank R, et al. Urolithiasis in pediatric patients: a single center study of incidence, clinical presentation and outcome. J Urol 2007;177(6):2300–5.
3. Dwyer ME, Krambeck AE, Bergstralh EJ, et al. Temporal trends in incidence of kidney stones among children: a 25-year population based study. J Urol 2012;188(1):247–52.
4. Routh JC, Graham DA, Nelson CP. Epidemiological trends in pediatric urolithiasis at United States free-standing pediatric hospitals. J Urol 2010;184(3): 1100–4.
5. Kokorowski PJ, Routh JC, Hubert KC, et al. Association of urolithiasis with systemic conditions among pediatric patients at children's hospitals. J Urol 2012; 188(Suppl 4):1618–22.
6. Kieran K, Giel DW, Morris BJ, et al. Pediatric urolithiasis–does body mass index influence stone presentation and treatment? J Urol 2010;184(Suppl 4):1810–5.
7. Lao M, Kogan BA, White MD, et al. High recurrence rate at 5-year followup in children after upper urinary tract stone surgery. J Urol 2014;191(2):440–4.

8. Tekin A, Tekgul S, Atsu N, et al. A study of the etiology of idiopathic calcium urolithiasis in children: hypocitruria is the most important risk factor. J Urol 2000; 164(1):162–5.

9. Penido MG, Srivastava T, Alon US. Pediatric primary urolithiasis: 12-year experience at a Midwestern Children's Hospital. J Urol 2013;189(4): 1493–7.

10. Gabrielsen JS, Laciak RJ, Frank EL, et al. Pediatric urinary stone composition in the United States. J Urol 2012;187(6):2182–7.

11. Coward RJ, Peters CJ, Duffy PG, et al. Epidemiology of paediatric renal stone disease in the UK. Arch Dis Child 2003;88(11):962–5.

12. Novak TE, Lakshmanan Y, Trock BJ, et al. Sex prevalence of pediatric kidney stone disease in the United States: an epidemiologic investigation. Urology 2009;74(1):104–7.

13. Routh JC, Graham DA, Nelson CP. Trends in imaging and surgical management of pediatric urolithiasis at American pediatric hospitals. J Urol 2010; 184(Suppl 4):1816–22.

14. Brenner D, Elliston C, Hall E, et al. Estimated risks of radiation-induced fatal cancer from pediatric CT. AJR Am J Roentgenol 2001;176(2):289–96.

15. Kuhns LR, Oliver WJ, Christodoulou E, et al. The predicted increased cancer risk associated with a single computed tomography examination for calculus detection in pediatric patients compared with the natural cancer incidence. Pediatr Emerg Care 2011;27(4):345–50.

16. Johnson EK, Faerber GJ, Roberts WW, et al. Are stone protocol computed tomography scans mandatory for children with suspected urinary calculi? Urology 2011;78(3):662–6.

17. Heidenreich A, Desgrandschamps F, Terrier F. Modern approach of diagnosis and management of acute flank pain: review of all imaging modalities. Eur Urol 2002;41(4):351–62.

18. Fulgham PF, Assimos DG, Pearle MS, et al. Clinical effectiveness protocols for imaging in the management of ureteral calculous disease: AUA technology assessment. J Urol 2013;189(4):1203–13.

19. Ray AA, Ghiculete D, Pace KT, et al. Limitations to ultrasound in the detection and measurement of urinary tract calculi. Urology 2010;76(2):295–300.

20. Palmer JS, Donaher ER, O'Riordan MA, et al. Diagnosis of pediatric urolithiasis: role of ultrasound and computerized tomography. J Urol 2005;174(4 Pt 1): 1413–6.

21. Lande MB, Varade W, Erkan E, et al. Role of urinary supersaturation in the evaluation of children with urolithiasis. Pediatr Nephrol 2005;20(4):491–4.

22. Kovacevic L, Wolfe-Christensen C, Edwards L, et al. From hypercalciuria to hypocitraturia–a shifting trend in pediatric urolithiasis? J Urol 2012; 188(Suppl 4):1623–7.

23. Tasian GE, Copelovitch L. Evaluation and Medical Management of Kidney Stones in Children. J Urol 2014. [Epub ahead of print].

24. Schaeffer AJ, Feng Z, Trock BJ, et al. Medical comorbidities associated with pediatric kidney stone disease. Urology 2011;77(1):195–9.

25. Preminger GM, Tiselius HG, Assimos DG, et al. 2007 guideline for the management of ureteral calculi. J Urol 2007;178(6):2418–34.

26. Smaldone MC, Cannon GM Jr, Wu HY, et al. Is ureteroscopy first line treatment for pediatric stone disease? J Urol 2007;178(5):2128–31 [discussion: 2131].

27. Kim SS, Kolon TF, Canter D, et al. Pediatric flexible ureteroscopic lithotripsy: the Children's Hospital of Philadelphia experience. J Urol 2008;180(6):2616–9 [discussion: 2619].

28. De Dominicis M, Matarazzo E, Capozza N, et al. Retrograde ureteroscopy for distal ureteric stone removal in children. BJU Int 2005;95(7):1049–52.

29. Deters LA, Dagrosa LM, Herrick BW, et al. Ultrasound guided ureteroscopy for the definitive management of ureteral stones: a randomized controlled trial. J Urol 2014. [Epub ahead of print].

30. Kokorowski PJ, Chow JS, Strauss KJ, et al. Prospective systematic intervention to reduce patient exposure to radiation during pediatric ureteroscopy. J Urol 2013;190(Suppl 4):1474–8.

31. Kocaoglu C, Ozkan KU. The effectiveness of 4.5F ultrathin semirigid ureteroscope in the management of ureteral stones in prepubertal children: is there a need for any ureteral dilatation? Urology 2014;84(1):202–5.

32. Herndon CD, Viamonte L, Joseph DB. Ureteroscopy in children: is there a need for ureteral dilation and postoperative stenting? J Pediatr Urol 2006;2(4):290–3.

33. Atar M, Sancaktutar AA, Penbegul N, et al. Comparison of a 4.5 F semi-rigid ureteroscope with a 7.5 F rigid ureteroscope in the treatment of ureteral stones in preschool-age children. Urol Res 2012; 40(6):733–8.

34. Tanriverdi O, Silay MS, Kendirci M, et al. Comparison of ureteroscopic procedures with rigid and semirigid ureteroscopes in pediatric population: does the caliber of instrument matter? Pediatr Surg Int 2010;26(7):733–8.

35. Schuster TG, Russell KY, Bloom DA, et al. Ureteroscopy for the treatment of urolithiasis in children. J Urol 2002;167(4):1813 [discussion: 1815–6].

36. Corcoran AT, Smaldone MC, Mally D, et al. When is prior ureteral stent placement necessary to access the upper urinary tract in prepubertal children? J Urol 2008;180(Suppl 4):1861–3 [discussion: 1863–4].

37. Mokhless I, Marzouk E, Thabet Ael D, et al. Ureteroscopy in infants and preschool age children: technique and preliminary results. Cent European J Urol 2012;65(1):30–2.

38. Singh A, Shah G, Young J, et al. Ureteral access sheath for the management of pediatric renal and ureteral stones: a single center experience. J Urol 2006;175(3 Pt 1):1080–2 [discussion: 1082].

39. Lallas CD, Auge BK, Raj GV, et al. Laser Doppler flowmetric determination of ureteral blood flow after ureteral access sheath placement. J Endourol 2002;16(8):583–90.

40. Wang HH, Huang L, Routh JC, et al. Use of the ureteral access sheath during ureteroscopy in children. J Urol 2011;186(Suppl 4):1728–33.

41. Traxer O, Thomas A. Prospective evaluation and classification of ureteral wall injuries resulting from insertion of a ureteral access sheath during retrograde intrarenal surgery. J Urol 2013;189(2):580–4.

42. Borboroglu PG, Amling CL, Schenkman NS, et al. Ureteral stenting after ureteroscopy for distal ureteral calculi: a multi-institutional prospective randomized controlled study assessing pain, outcomes and complications. J Urol 2001;166(5):1651–7.

43. Haleblian G, Kijvikai K, de la Rosette J, et al. Ureteral stenting and urinary stone management: a systematic review. J Urol 2008;179(2):424–30.

44. Atar M, Bodakci MN, Sancaktutar AA, et al. Comparison of pneumatic and laser lithotripsy in the treatment of pediatric ureteral stones. J Pediatr Urol 2013;9(3):308–12.

45. Jeon SS, Hyun JH, Lee KS. A comparison of holmium:YAG laser with Lithoclast lithotripsy in ureteral calculi fragmentation. Int J Urol 2005;12(6):544–7.

46. Afshar K, McLorie G, Papanikolaou F, et al. Outcome of small residual stone fragments following shock wave lithotripsy in children. J Urol 2004;172(4 Pt 2):1600–3.

47. Minevich E, Defoor W, Reddy P, et al. Ureteroscopy is safe and effective in prepubertal children. J Urol 2005;174(1):276–9 [discussion: 279].

48. Bassiri A, Ahmadnia H, Darabi MR, et al. Transureteral lithotripsy in pediatric practice. J Endourol 2002;16(4):257–60.

49. Raza A, Smith G, Moussa S, et al. Ureteroscopy in the management of pediatric urinary tract calculi. J Endourol 2005;19(2):151–8.

50. al Busaidy SS, Prem AR, Medhat M. Paediatric ureteroscopy for ureteric calculi: a 4-year experience. Br J Urol 1997;80(5):797–801.

51. Satar N, Zeren S, Bayazit Y, et al. Rigid ureteroscopy for the treatment of ureteral calculi in children. J Urol 2004;172(1):298–300.

52. Hubert KC, Palmer JS. Passive dilation by ureteral stenting before ureteroscopy: eliminating the need for active dilation. J Urol 2005;174(3):1079–80 [discussion: 1080].

53. Nerli RB, Patil SM, Guntaka AK, et al. Flexible ureteroscopy for upper ureteral calculi in children. J Endourol 2011;25(4):579–82.

54. Tanaka ST, Makari JH, Pope JC, et al. Pediatric ureteroscopic management of intrarenal calculi. J Urol 2008;180(5):2150–3 [discussion: 2153–4].

55. Dave S, Khoury AE, Braga L, et al. Single-institutional study on role of ureteroscopy and retrograde intrarenal surgery in treatment of pediatric renal calculi. Urology 2008;72(5):1018–21.

56. Dogan HS, Onal B, Satar N, et al. Factors affecting complication rates of ureteroscopic lithotripsy in children: results of multi-institutional retrospective analysis by Pediatric Stone Disease Study Group of Turkish Pediatric Urology Society. J Urol 2011;186(3):1035–40.

57. Tiryaki T, Azili MN, Ozmert S. Ureteroscopy for treatment of ureteral stones in children: factors influencing the outcome. Urology 2013;81(5):1047–51.

58. Erkurt B, Caskurlu T, Atis G, et al. Treatment of renal stones with flexible ureteroscopy in preschool age children. Urolithiasis 2014;42(3):241–5.

59. Moltzahn F, Haeni K, Birkhauser FD, et al. Peri-interventional antibiotic prophylaxis only vs continuous low-dose antibiotic treatment in patients with JJ stents: a prospective randomised trial analysing the effect on urinary tract infections and stent-related symptoms. BJU Int 2013;111(2):289–95.

60. Woodside JR, Stevens GF, Stark GL, et al. Percutaneous stone removal in children. J Urol 1985;134(6):1166–7.

61. Traxer O, Smith TG 3rd, Pearle MS, et al. Renal parenchymal injury after standard and mini percutaneous nephrostolithotomy. J Urol 2001;165(5):1693–5.

62. Al-Kandari AM, Jabbour M, Anderson A, et al. Comparative study of degree of renal trauma between Amplatz sequential fascial dilation and balloon dilation during percutaneous renal surgery in an animal model. Urology 2007;69(3):586–9.

63. Samad L, Qureshi S, Zaidi Z. Does percutaneous nephrolithotomy in children cause significant renal scarring? J Pediatr Urol 2007;3(1):36–9.

64. Dawaba MS, Shokeir AA, Hafez A, et al. Percutaneous nephrolithotomy in children: early and late anatomical and functional results. J Urol 2004;172(3):1078–81.

65. Okhunov Z, Friedlander JI, George AK, et al. S.T.O.N.E. nephrolithometry: novel surgical classification system for kidney calculi. Urology 2013;81(6):1154–9.

66. Thomas K, Smith NC, Hegarty N, et al. The Guy's stone score–grading the complexity of percutaneous nephrolithotomy procedures. Urology 2011;78(2):277–81.

67. Park J, Hong B, Park T, et al. Effectiveness of noncontrast computed tomography in evaluation of residual

stones after percutaneous nephrolithotomy. J Endourol 2007;21(7):684–7.

68. Dagli M, Ramchandani P. Percutaneous nephrostomy: technical aspects and indications. Semin Intervent Radiol 2011;28(4):424–37.

69. Watterson JD, Soon S, Jana K. Access related complications during percutaneous nephrolithotomy: urology versus radiology at a single academic institution. J Urol 2006;176(1):142–5.

70. El-Assmy AM, Shokeir AA, Mohsen T, et al. Renal access by urologist or radiologist for percutaneous nephrolithotomy–is it still an issue? J Urol 2007; 178(3 Pt 1):916–20 [discussion: 920].

71. Lashley DB, Fuchs EF. Urologist-acquired renal access for percutaneous renal surgery. Urology 1998; 51(6):927–31.

72. Bird VG, Fallon B, Winfield HN. Practice patterns in the treatment of large renal stones. J Endourol 2003;17(6):355–63.

73. Onal B, Dogan HS, Satar N, et al. Factors affecting complication rates of percutaneous nephrolithotomy in children: results of a multi-institutional retrospective analysis by the Turkish pediatric urology society. J Urol 2014;191(3):777–82.

74. McAllister M, Lim K, Torrey R, et al. Intercostal vessels and nerves are at risk for injury during supracostal percutaneous nephrostolithotomy. J Urol 2011; 185(1):329–34.

75. Anand A, Kumar R, Dogra PN, et al. Safety and efficacy of a superior caliceal puncture in pediatric percutaneous nephrolithotomy. J Endourol 2010; 24(11):1725–8.

76. Guven S, Frattini A, Onal B, et al. Percutaneous nephrolithotomy in children in different age groups: data from the Clinical Research Office of the Endourological Society (CROES) Percutaneous Nephrolithotomy Global Study. BJU Int 2013; 111(1):148–56.

77. Kumar R, Anand A, Saxena V, et al. Safety and efficacy of PCNL for management of staghorn calculi in pediatric patients. J Pediatr Urol 2011; 7(3):248–51.

78. Khairy Salem H, Morsi HA, Omran A, et al. Tubeless percutaneous nephrolithotomy in children. J Pediatr Urol 2007;3(3):235–8.

79. Bilen CY, Gunay M, Ozden E, et al. Tubeless mini percutaneous nephrolithotomy in infants and preschool children: a preliminary report. J Urol 2010; 184(6):2498–502.

80. Bader MJ, Gratzke C, Seitz M, et al. The "all-seeing needle": initial results of an optical puncture system confirming access in percutaneous nephrolithotomy. Eur Urol 2011;59(6):1054–9.

81. Singla M, Srivastava A, Kapoor R, et al. Aggressive approach to staghorn calculi-safety and efficacy of multiple tracts percutaneous nephrolithotomy. Urology 2008;71(6):1039–42.

82. Miller NL, Matlaga BR, Lingeman JE. Techniques for fluoroscopic percutaneous renal access. J Urol 2007;178(1):15–23.

83. Jackman SV, Hedican SP, Peters CA, et al. Percutaneous nephrolithotomy in infants and preschool age children: experience with a new technique. Urology 1998;52(4):697–701.

84. Sabnis RB, Ganesamoni R, Sarpal R. Miniperc: what is its current status? Curr Opin Urol 2012; 22(2):129–33.

85. Mishra S, Sharma R, Garg C, et al. Prospective comparative study of miniperc and standard PNL for treatment of 1 to 2 cm size renal stone. BJU Int 2011;108(6):896–9 [discussion: 899–900].

86. Guven S, Istanbulluoglu O, Gul U, et al. Successful percutaneous nephrolithotomy in children: multicenter study on current status of its use, efficacy and complications using Clavien classification. J Urol 2011;185(4):1419–24.

87. Zeng G, Zhao Z, Wan S, et al. Comparison of children versus adults undergoing mini-percutaneous nephrolithotomy: large-scale analysis of a single institution. PLoS One 2013;8(6):e66850.

88. Desai MR, Sharma R, Mishra S, et al. Single-step percutaneous nephrolithotomy (microperc): the initial clinical report. J Urol 2011;186(1):140–5.

89. De Sio M, Autorino R, Quarto G, et al. Modified supine versus prone position in percutaneous nephrolithotomy for renal stones treatable with a single percutaneous access: a prospective randomized trial. Eur Urol 2008;54(1):196–202.

90. Lawrentschuk N, Pan D, Grills R, et al. Outcome from percutaneous nephrolithotomy in patients with spinal cord injury, using a single-stage dilator for access. BJU Int 2005;96(3):379–84.

91. Mor Y, Elmasry YE, Kellett MJ, et al. The role of percutaneous nephrolithotomy in the management of pediatric renal calculi. J Urol 1997;158(3 Pt 2): 1319–21.

92. Badawy H, Salama A, Eissa M, et al. Percutaneous management of renal calculi: experience with percutaneous nephrolithotomy in 60 children. J Urol 1999;162(5):1710–3.

93. Al-Shammari AM, Al-Otaibi K, Leonard MP, et al. Percutaneous nephrolithotomy in the pediatric population. J Urol 1999;162(5):1721–4.

94. Zeren S, Satar N, Bayazit Y, et al. Percutaneous nephrolithotomy in the management of pediatric renal calculi. J Endourol 2002;16(2):75–8.

95. Rizvi SA, Naqvi SA, Hussain Z, et al. Management of pediatric urolithiasis in Pakistan: experience with 1,440 children. J Urol 2003;169(2):634–7.

96. Desai MR, Kukreja RA, Patel SH, et al. Percutaneous nephrolithotomy for complex pediatric renal calculus disease. J Endourol 2004;18(1):23–7.

97. Salah MA, Toth C, Khan AM, et al. Percutaneous nephrolithotomy in children: experience with 138

cases in a developing country. World J Urol 2004;22(4):277–80.

98.. Raza A, Turna B, Smith G, et al. Pediatric urolithiasis: 15 years of local experience with minimally invasive endourological management of pediatric calculi. J Urol 2005;174(2):682–5.

99. Shokeir AA, Sheir KZ, El-Nahas AR, et al. Treatment of renal stones in children: a comparison between percutaneous nephrolithotomy and shock wave lithotripsy. J Urol 2006;176(2):706–10.

100. Bilen CY, Kocak B, Kitirci G, et al. Percutaneous nephrolithotomy in children: lessons learned in 5 years at a single institution. J Urol 2007;177(5): 1867–71.

101. Roth CC, Donovan BO, Adams JM, et al. Use of second look nephroscopy in children undergoing percutaneous nephrolithotomy. J Urol 2009; 181(2):796–800.

102. Nouralizadeh A, Basiri A, Javaherforooshzadeh A, et al. Experience of percutaneous nephrolithotomy using adult-size instruments in children less than 5 years old. J Pediatr Urol 2009;5(5):351–4.

103. Unsal A, Resorlu B, Kara C, et al. Safety and efficacy of percutaneous nephrolithotomy in infants, preschool age, and older children with different sizes of instruments. Urology 2010;76(1):247–52.

104. Veeratterapillay R, Shaw MB, Williams R, et al. Safety and efficacy of percutaneous nephrolithotomy for the treatment of paediatric urolithiasis. Ann R Coll Surg Engl 2012;94(8):588–92.

105. Bhageria A, Nayak B, Seth A, et al. Paediatric percutaneous nephrolithotomy: single-centre 10-year experience. J Pediatr Urol 2013;9(4):472–5.

106. Yan X, Al-Hayek S, Gan W, et al. Minimally invasive percutaneous nephrolithotomy in preschool age children with kidney calculi (including stones induced by melamine-contaminated milk powder). Pediatr Surg Int 2012;28(10):1021–4.

107. Wah TM, Kidger L, Kennish S, et al. MINI PCNL in a pediatric population. Cardiovasc Intervent Radiol 2013;36(1):249–54.

108. Goyal NK, Goel A, Sankhwar SN, et al. A critical appraisal of complications of percutaneous nephrolithotomy in paediatric patients using adult instruments. BJU Int 2014;113(5):801–10.

109. Samad L, Aquil S, Zaidi Z. Paediatric percutaneous nephrolithotomy: setting new frontiers. BJU Int 2006;97(2):359–63.

110. Etemadian M, Maghsoudi R, Shadpour P, et al. Pediatric percutaneous nephrolithotomy using adult sized instruments: our experience. Urol J 2012; 9(2):465–71.

111. Uygun I, Okur MH, Aydogdu B, et al. Efficacy and safety of endoscopic laser lithotripsy for urinary stone treatment in children. Urol Res 2012;40(6): 751–5.

112. Yucel S, Akin Y, Kol A, et al. Experience on semirigid ureteroscopy and pneumatic lithotripsy in children at a single center. World J Urol 2011;29(6): 719–23.

Laparoscopic Orchiopexy and Varicocelectomy
Is There Really an Advantage?

Ronnie G. Fine, MD[a],*, Israel Franco, MD[b]

KEYWORDS

- Laparoscopy • Varicocele • Varicocelectomy • Undescended testis • Orchiopexy • Adolescent
- Pediatric • Surgical technique

KEY POINTS

- Laparoscopy is the gold standard diagnostic modality for a nonpalpable testis.
- Once an abdominal testis is detected, one must determine whether the testis can be brought into the scrotum in 1 or 2 stages.
- There is controversy as to whether a testicular remnant should be excised and if a contralateral orchiopexy is needed.
- Indications for varicocelectomy in an adolescent are left testicular hypotrophy (>10%–20%), abnormal semen analysis or pain.
- Critics of the laparoscopic procedure have argued that this does not provide superior outcomes while introducing the significant risks to intra-abdominal contents associated with laparoscopy.

INTRODUCTION: LAPAROSCOPIC ORCHIOPEXY – WHAT IS THE ADVANTAGE?

Unilateral or bilateral cryptorchidism is found in 4% of newborns[1] and 0.8% to 2% of 1-year-old boys, and 20% to 35% of those are nonpalpable testes.[2,3] A testis that has not descended by 6 months of age is unlikely to descend; therefore, surgery should be considered.[4] The cryptorchid testis may be difficult to palpate in an awake and uncooperative child or an obese child with a large suprapubic fat pad. In rare instances, a sonogram may be helpful to plan the surgical approach but in general is of little to no value. A truly nonpalpable testis may represent an intra-abdominal undescended testis (vanishing testis), which is one that had atrophied before evaluation, or testicular agenesis/dysgenesis. The atrophic testis can be found in the scrotal position and is thought to be a prenatal event in a descended or descending testis. In that case, the internal ring is usually closed, and the testicular vessels are seen entering it, along with the vas deferens. It is common to palpate a testicular remnant (nubbin) in the upper scrotum. A vanishing testis may also be represented by blind-ending vessels in an intra-abdominal position. Early testicular atrophy is usually accompanied by contralateral testicular compensatory hypertrophy, a finding that provides a clue to the true diagnosis.[5] Agenesis or dysgenesis of a testis is uncommon and may be associated with disordered sexual differentiation or even absence of the contralateral kidney.

A cryptorchid testis is at a higher risk (risk ratio, 2.5–8) of malignancy development than a scrotal testis.[6–8] These patients have a slightly higher risk of testicular cancer in the contralateral testis as well.[9] Orchiopexy before puberty may significantly

R. Fine has nothing to disclose; Allergen consultant and clinical researcher, Astellas consultant and clinical researcher (I. Franco).
a Department of Urology, Long Island Jewish Hospital, 270-05 76th Ave, New Hyde Park, NY 11040, USA;
b Department of Urology, New York Medical College, 40 Sunshine Cottage Rd, Valhalla, NY 10595, USA
* Corresponding author.
E-mail address: rog2003@gmail.com

Urol Clin N Am 42 (2015) 19–29
http://dx.doi.org/10.1016/j.ucl.2014.09.003
0094-0143/15/$ – see front matter © 2015 Elsevier Inc. All rights reserved.

urologic.theclinics.com

decrease the risk of malignancy later in life.[10] Additionally, there is an association between cryptorchidism and decreased fertility caused by testicular dysfunction, particularly in bilateral cases.[11] An inguinal hernia is often associated with the undescended testis and is another cause for concern. Finally, testicular torsion would be difficult to diagnose in an abdominal testis and would increase the risk of testicular loss.

The role of laparoscopy in the management of a nonpalpable testicle is 2-fold. Diagnostic laparoscopy was first described by Cortesi in 1976, and has been accepted as the gold standard for the diagnosis of a nonpalpable testicle.[12] The preferred method of treating an intra-abdominal testis is no longer controversial. The combined inguinal/retroperitoneal open approach has been largely replaced by laparoscopy, which was first described in the 1990s.[13,14] In capable hands, the laparoscopic approach has equivalent or superior outcomes as the open one with regard to testicular viability and scrotal position. It also provides the advantages of the minimally invasive approach, with decreased postoperative pain and scarring.[15] There is still debate regarding the need to divide the testicular vessels in high intra-abdominal testes (Fowler Stephen's approach),[16] and whether to do that in 1 or 2 stages.[17]

Diagnostic laparoscopy may show the absence of one or both testes. A testicular nubbin can be excised via an open approach (scrotal or inguinal) and rarely laparoscopically. It is controversial whether it is necessary to remove a testicular nubbin, as it has not been associated with malignancy.[6,18] The decision to perform a scrotal orchiopexy in the case of a solitary contralateral testis is one that should be made after discussion with the parents preoperatively and is based on the surgeon's preference.[19]

Cost analysis finds that the use of laparoscopy does not increase the cost of the procedure when compared with the open approach if it is done with reusable instrumentation and operating room time is low (**Fig. 1**).[20]

INDICATIONS

- A nonpalpable abdominal testis
- Recurrent iatrogenic cryptorchidism (redo orchiopexy)
- Option: High canalicular/peeping testes
- Unusual cases: bilateral orchiopexy, abdominal wall defects, polyorchidism, splenogonadal fusion, and transverse testicular ectopia[21]

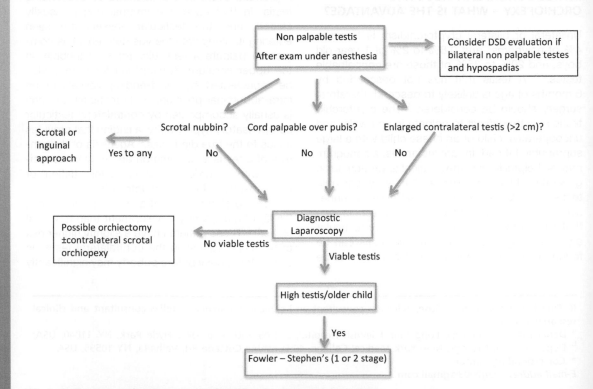

Fig. 1. Evaluation and management algorithm for a nonpalpable testis.

The most definitive method of evaluating and potentially treating a nonpalpable testis is laparoscopically, as imaging modalities have repeatedly show low sensitivity and specificity for accurately locating an undescended testicle.[7,22,23] A physical examination performed by a trained specialist of a nonobese child, awake or under anesthesia, is highly accurate in differentiating a palpable versus a nonpalpable testis. Once the testis is determined to be nonpalpable, a diagnostic laparoscopy is performed to identify its location and viability.

A laparoscopic approach is also possible in cases in which the initial orchiopexy failed to result in a scrotal position of the testis. A reoperative inguinal approach to a recurrent undescended testis may be limited by scarring and inability to gain additional length through a groin incision. The laparoscopic approach provides the benefit of accessing virginal tissues with the potential of mobilizing the testicular vessels proximally.[24,25]

The use of laparoscopy in palpable inguinal testes has been examined. He and colleagues[26] and Riquelme and colleagues[27] reported on a series of 103 and 30 testes, respectively, in which they used laparoscopy in the management of palpable canalicular testes with success rates equivalent to an open technique and with the advantages of laparoscopy.

CONTRAINDICATIONS

- Extensive prior retroperitoneal or abdominal surgery
- Prior peritonitis
- Abdominal wall infection
- Large hernia
- Cardiopulmonary disease
- Coagulopathy

PROCEDURE
Positioning

- Position the patient at the end of the table, as the child is typically young and their torso is short, so the surgeon will be at the upper portion of the table facing the patient's feet and on the left of the patient (if right handed).
- Do not elevate the pelvis with a rolled towel, as that will decrease the intra-abdominal working space.

Preparation

- Prepare from xiphoid to the midthighs.
- Catheterize the bladder on the field with a feeding tube.

Detailed Steps

- Place a camera port at the umbilicus.
- Inspect the abdomen. Abort the case if a testis is not found intra-abdominally. A nubbin may be excised at this time.
- Look for a vas if the testis is not readily identified. In some instances, the testis may be deep in the pelvis, and looking for the vas at the takeoff of the seminal vesicles will lead to identification of the testicle.
- Add 2 lateral ports if a viable testis is found. Consider using a 5-mm port for the camera. This will come in handy later to pass a 5-mm trocar through the scrotum (**Fig. 2**).
- For a peeping testis, place traction on the testis itself and do not handle the epididymis (**Fig. 3**).
- Ensure that the epididymis and vas do not loop into the inguinal canal (if you cannot be sure that the epididymis and vas are safe, do not hesitate to make a groin incision at this point if needed).
- If the vas and epididymis are clear, transect the gubernaculum (if it bleeds you likely cut the epididymis and not pure gubernaculum).
- Lift the peritoneum and dissect medially over the median umbilical ligament and then lift the peritoneum off the bladder, leaving a cuff of peritoneum away from the vas (**Fig. 4**).
- Make the lateral wall dissection as high as possible along the lateral edge of the psoas (**Fig. 5**).
- Come across the peritoneum over the gonadal vessels at this point (trying to free the peritoneum when the testis is on tension leads to a high probability that the gonadal vessels will be inadvertently transected, potentially leading to delayed bleeding).
- Continue the dissection down the peritoneum to the root of the small bowel mesentery.
- Mobilize the bladder off the pubic bone medial to the median umbilical ligament (ensure that

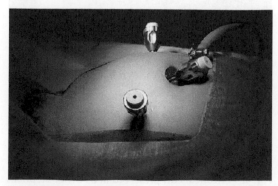

Fig. 2. Trocar placement.

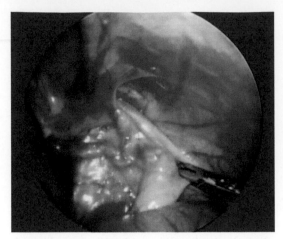

Fig. 3. Traction on the testicle to transect the gubernaculum.

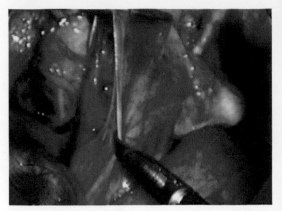

Fig. 5. Peritoneal edge.

the feeding tube is in the bladder and the bladder is empty).

- Use a dissector (Maryland) to push over the pubic bone while inverting the scrotum, and feel for the thinnest area, which is the external inguinal ring.
- Push the dissector through the anterior abdominal wall (a pop will be felt).
- Make an incision in the scrotum and create the subdartos pouch.
- Push the dissector through the scrotal incision and back load a 5-mm trocar over the dissector and push into the abdomen (**Fig. 6**).
- Use a toothed grasper and bring this through the 5-mm trocar and hand the testis to the toothed grasper with the other hand. (Make sure that the testis is grasped and not the epididymis or vas.)

- Bring the testis through the neo-canal. (Pull the testis into the trocar as far as possible; this will make the testis more elliptical and will facilitate the removal of the testis through the canal.)
- As soon as the testis is in the field, grab the testis with a toothed forceps and then place your anchoring sutures.
- Deflate the abdomen at this time and check the testis position. (With the abdomen inflated, the testis typically will sit much higher in the scrotum.)
- If there is not enough length and the testis is in an unsatisfactory position, a Fowler-Stephens orchiopexy can be performed at this time.
- A clip applier can be brought into the field and the vessels clipped and transected.
- Once the testis has been anchored with the abdomen deflated, reinflate the abdomen and inspect for bleeding that may have occurred. Make sure that the ureters have not been elevated or kinked (**Fig. 7**).
- Close each trocar port.

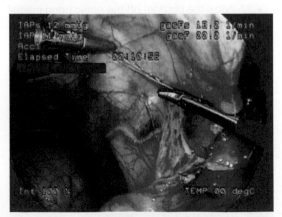

Fig. 4. Peritoneal cuff preserved in a Fowler-Stephens case.

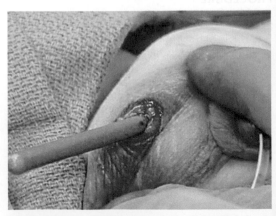

Fig. 6. Dissector placed through the neo-canal.

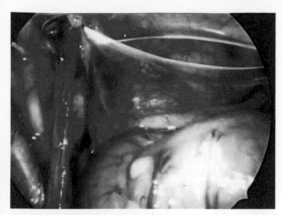

Fig. 7. Testis exiting new ring.

COMPLICATIONS AND MANAGEMENT

- Testicular atrophy
- Recurrence
- Vascular injury
- Bladder injury

Testicular Atrophy

- Atrophy may be evident on physical examination at the second postoperative visit, generally 6 months after the procedure, but in some instances it may not be evident until 1 year from surgery. Some have advocated the use of a sonogram to confirm testicular viability, but in prepubertal testes it can be difficult to get good flow curves, and the delayed examination 1 year or later is the best test for viability. The risk of atrophy, which is irreversible, drives many practitioners to approach bilateral orchiopexy in a staged approach.
- Single-stage Fowler-Stephen's orchiopexy has the highest rate of atrophy (3%–22%), whereas a vessel-sparing procedure had the lowest atrophy rates (0%–4%).[28–32]
- A long looping vas was found to be a risk factor for testicular atrophy in cases of laparoscopic second-stage orchiopexy, presumably because of inability to preserve collateral vassal blood supply adequately.[33]

Recurrent Cryptorchidism

- This complication, which is reported in 0% to 19% of laparoscopic orchiopexy series is caused by insufficient mobilization of the testis or inadequate testicular fixation and often requires a secondary procedure.[28,32,34,35] This procedure should be attempted at least 6 to 12 months after the initial procedure to

allow for maximal healing and possible testicular descent in the interim.

Bladder Injury

- This injury occurs during the creation of the transperitoneal tunnel for the undescended testis between the bladder and the obliterated umbilical ligament. It may result in significant morbidity if it is not identified intraoperatively; therefore, one must maintain a high index of suspicion.
- This risk may be minimized by emptying the bladder before the creation of the tunnel and aspiration of the bladder. It is also helpful to perform extensive dissection lateral to the bladder to enable visualization of the bladder edge.
- This injury should be suspected when there is difficulty creating the tunnel or any degree of hematuria is present; however, hematuria may be absent in some cases. Cystoscopy should be performed to confirm the injury. Alternatively, if the diagnosis is delayed, a cystogram can provide the diagnostic information.
- Management of this transperitoneal injury requires bladder repair, which can be done laparoscopically, depending on the practitioner's level of confidence. The bladder must be decompressed with a catheter after the repair to facilitate recovery; however, the duration is not agreed upon.[36]

Vascular Injury

- Injury to the femoral vessels during passage of the dissector into the scrotum is a potentially catastrophic event. This event can be reliably avoided by creating the neo-canal from lateral to medial and by dissection of the space between the bladder and the obliterated umbilical vessels down to the pubic bone in preparation for the blind advancement of the dissector.[37]
- Injury to iliac vessels during laparoscopic mobilization of the testis
- Inadvertent avulsion of the testicular vessels during delivery of the testis into the scrotum may be caused by excessive traction on the testis when at the time the surgeon is focused on the scrotal aspect of the procedure and does not have intra-abdominal visualization. Furthermore, the vessels may have been avulsed but in spasm, making recognition of this injury more difficult. Therefore, it is advised to incise the peritoneum before delivering the testis, as injury to the vessels will be readily evident. It is recommended that the

surgeon, not the assistant, be the person holding the testis when the testis is on traction and dissection of the vessels is occurring, because they can feel the tension in the cord structure during the dissection. It is important to have a high level of suspicion for such a complication to address it intraoperatively by controlling the vessels.

Complications associated with laparoscopy are rare but must be discussed (hypercapnia, injury to intra-abdominal organs, port site hernia, delayed bowel obstruction caused by adhesions).

POSTOPERATIVE CARE

Laparoscopic orchiopexy is usually performed on an outpatient basis. Patients are discharged from the postanesthesia care unit and are seen 1 to 2 week postoperatively and then at 3 and 6 months postoperatively.

Postoperative care and restrictions are essentially identical as for an inguinal orchiopexy and are practitioner dependent. Restrictions may involve avoidance of heavy lifting and straddle toys for several weeks; however, the role of activity restrictions has not been systematically addressed.

FOLLOW-UP AND CLINICAL IMPLICATIONS

A minimum of 12-month follow-up is needed to evaluate the success of an orchiopexy. Testicular atrophy or recurrent cryptorchidism should be evident within that timeframe in most patients. Testicular atrophy is generally apparent within 6 months, but sometimes 12 months is needed for Fowler-Stephens orchiopexies. Follow-up consists of a physical examination, which is a good indicator of testicular viability. The undescended testis is usually smaller than the contralateral descended testis at the time of surgery, and long-term follow-up showed that the size discrepancy is persistent into adulthood even when it is well vascularized.[38]

OUTCOMES

Most published series consider a successful laparoscopic orchiopexy one that results in a viable testicle and a mid to low scrotal position. Testicular atrophy or recurrent cryptorchidism has been reported in 0% to 35% of laparoscopic orchiopexy series.[22,28,32,34] Performing a Fowler-Stephens orchiopexy or a redo procedure significantly increases the risk of atrophy. One-step Fowler-Stephens laparoscopic orchiopexy series report a higher rate of testicular atrophy

(3%–22%) versus the 2-step Fowler-Stephens procedure (0%–15%).[21] In a report of long-term outcome in 12 patients that underwent a 2-stage Fowler-Stephens orchiopexy, 83% of patients had satisfactory results more than 10 years postoperatively.[38]

CURRENT CONTROVERSIES AND FUTURE CONSIDERATIONS

The high rate of successfully managed intra-abdominal testes that are corrected laparoscopically has allowed this approach to become the standard of care. The main controversy is whether it is possible to avoid transection of the gonadal vessels in all cases of high abdominal testis.[39] Others have questioned the benefit of performing the Fowler-Stephens approach in 2 stages rather than one, citing similar results in the single stage when the vasal vessels are properly preserved.[16,17,40]

SUMMARY

- Laparoscopy is the gold standard for the diagnosis of a nonpalpable testis.
- Once an abdominal testis is detected, one must determine whether the testis can be brought into the scrotum in 1 or 2 stages.
- A vessel transection approach to achieve adequate length (Fowler-Stephens approach) may be performed in 1 or 2 stages. The 2-stage approach has a slightly lower risk of testicular atrophy.
- The most common complications are testicular atrophy and persistent or recurrent cryptorchidism.
- There is controversy as to whether a testicular remnant should be excised and if a contralateral orchiopexy is needed

INTRODUCTION
The Adolescent Varicocele

It has been estimated that 4% to 15% of adolescents harbor a grade 2 to 3 varicocele.[41–43] For the most part, the patients are asymptomatic and the varicocele is diagnosed on a routine physical examination. Because of their young age, the patients do not present with infertility. They rarely complain of pain, with the exception of long-distance runners, in our experience. The patients may present with a testicular size discrepancy in which there is a loss of left testicular volume. This size differential is attributed to abnormal testicular development in the presence of a varicocele; however, this is debatable, as many patients experience left testicular catch-up growth with observation alone.[44–46] It is also debatable whether a varicocele in an adolescent represents a risk for progressive deterioration in gonadal function, requiring early correction.[47] Most adolescents are not referred for a semen analysis by their pediatric urologist despite it being the cornerstone of the workup of an adult with a varicocele (Author's own data, Unpublished data).

Microsurgical, laparoscopic, open (Palomo), and endovascular sclerotherapy techniques are being used in the treatment of a varicocele. Reviews within the adult literature have concluded that the microsurgical subinguinal approach had superior results in terms of pregnancy rates and complications such as recurrence and hydrocele formation.[48,49] However, when analyzing the pediatric population, laparoscopic varicocelectomy had equivalent outcomes to open techniques.[50,51]

The main variation within this approach is whether hot or cold ligation of the testicular vessels is done[52,53] and whether the testicular artery and lymphatics are spared.[54,55] Several investigators have reported results of laparoendoscopic single-site surgery with satisfactory results.[56–58] The laparoscopic approach has gained traction as pediatric urologists have become increasingly facile with laparoscopic techniques. Laparoscopic magnification facilitates the dissection of the vein away from the artery and lymphatics, and access to the suprainguinal testicular vessels allows for increased efficiency in the operating room and decreased surgical costs.

Indications

Indications for a varicocelectomy include persistent or progressive left-sided testicular hypotrophy, abnormal sperm count or abnormal sperm motility, or pain attributable to a varicocele. Most varicoceles can be approached laparoscopically, particularly when there was previous groin surgery, such as an inguinal hernia repair. There is some benefit to this approach when treating bilateral varicoceles if additional incisions are avoided. The choice of approach depends on the surgeon's and the patient's preference.

Contraindications

- Extensive prior retroperitoneal or abdominal surgery
- Prior peritonitis
- Abdominal wall infection
- Large hernia
- Cardiopulmonary disease
- Coagulopathy

PROCEDURE
Preparation

- Have the patient void before going into the operating room to avoid bladder catheterization at the time of the procedure.
- Prepare the patient from xiphoid to upper thighs, lateral to iliac spines, include penis scrotum

Positioning

- The patient is positioned in a slight Trendelenburg position.

Detailed Steps

- Make umbilical trocar incision and insufflate the abdominal cavity.
- Place your trocars under direct vision. Place camera port in the midpoint between the pubis and the umbilicus; second working port at the level of the umbilicus, lateral to the rectus muscle, ipsilateral to the varicocele (**Fig. 8**).
- Identify the gonadal vessels (**Fig. 9**). Make an incision in the peritoneum lateral to the gonadal vessels, and elevate the peritoneum to allow for pneumodissection.
- Incise the peritoneum medially up to the edge of the iliac vessels.
- Isolate the largest vessel (typically the artery is adjacent to this vessel).
- If the artery is going to be preserved, then isolate this at this time. (The less manipulation around the artery the more likely you will see the pulsations of the artery; use of a laparoscopic Doppler can help in identification of the artery as well.)
- Grasp the largest vessel and separate the adventitia at this time; within this adventitia you will find most of the lymphatics that can be preserved (**Fig. 10**).

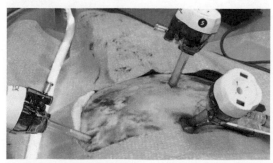

Fig. 8. View from the head toward the feet. Camera is placed in the lower midline port.

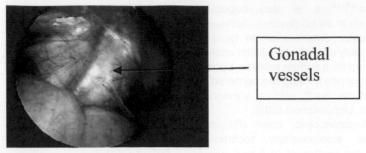

Fig. 9. Left gonadal vessels.

- Once the vein or veins are isolated from the lymphatics, clip the vessels and cut them. (The artery can be taken with the veins; **Fig. 11.**)
- Inspect for residual veins and if present clip them.
- Deflate the abdomen and inspect for bleeding.

COMPLICATIONS AND MANAGEMENT

- Hydrocele formation
- Recurrence
- Nerve injury
- Testicular atrophy

Hydrocele

- Hydrocele is the most common complication in procedures in which the artery and lymphatics are not spared. It was noted in some series in up to 25% to 43% of all cases; however, only a third of hydroceles did not resolve and required intervention.[55]
- Hydrocele formation in lymphatic- and artery-sparing procedures is rare, at 0% to 4%, which is comparable to that of the microsurgical subinguinal approach.[50,51]

- Many hydroceles appear in a delayed fashion, 6 to 36 months postoperatively, and patients may be lost to follow-up. This finding may result in underrecognition of the true rate of hydrocele formation.
- Initial management of a postoperative hydrocele requires observation, as most will resolve. A persistent, growing, or bothersome hydrocele will require sclerosis or a formal hydrocelectomy.

Recurrence or Persistence

- Meta-analysis shows recurrence or persistence in 4% to 5% of cases.[49–51]
- This complication is more commonly associated with artery and lymphatics preservation as the likelihood of a missed varicocele increases.
- Recurrence may be detected several years postoperatively, stressing the importance of long-term follow-up in these patients.

Nerve Injury

- Nerve injury is reported in 0% to 4% of cases. It is usually reported several days postoperatively when the patient notices numbness or

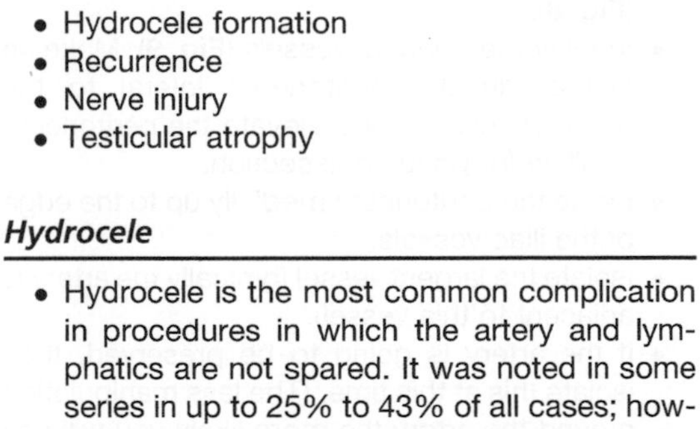

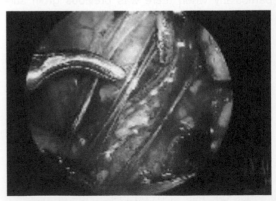

Fig. 10. The largest vein is dissected away from the artery and lymphatics.

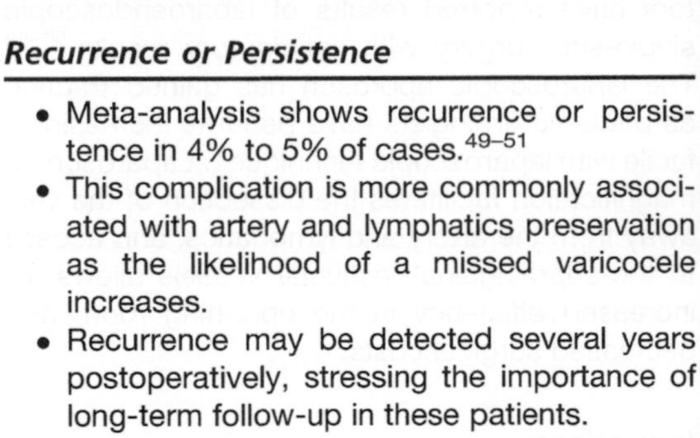

Fig. 11. The vein is clipped and cut. All lymphatics and the artery are preserved.

paresthesia in the genitofemoral nerve distribution (ipsilateral anterior thigh).
- The risk is small and may be diminished by avoidance of electrocautery.[52,53]
- Observation and reassurance is recommended, as the symptoms resolve within 6 to 9 months.

Testicular Atrophy

- Testicular atrophy is a rare complication associated with prior inguinal surgery in which collateral blood supply to the testis was damaged.
- In these cases, the testicular artery should be spared.

Complications associated with laparoscopy are rare but must be discussed (hypercapnia, injury to intra-abdominal organs, port site hernia, delayed bowel obstruction due to adhesions).

POSTOPERATIVE CARE

Laparoscopic varicocelectomy is performed on an outpatient basis. Patients are discharged from the postanesthesia care unit and are seen 1 to 2 week postoperatively and then at 3, 6, and 12 months postoperatively.

Postoperative care and restrictions are essentially identical to those for open varicocelectomy and are practitioner dependent.

REPORTING, FOLLOW-UP, AND CLINICAL IMPLICATIONS

- The first postoperative visit within 1 to 3 weeks includes a physical examination.
- A repeat semen analysis is optional if a baseline one was done.
- Scrotal sonogram may be used to assess for testicular size difference and catch-up growth as well as residual/recurrent varicocele.
- Sparing of the artery and lymphatics leads to increased risk of residual or recurrent varicocele and may warrant a repeat procedure.
- If there are no complications, there is a second postoperative visit at 6 months and a third visit at 1 year.
- Long-term follow-up is recommended to identify varicocele recurrence.

OUTCOMES

Outcomes of laparoscopic varicocelectomy are reported to be similar to those of the Palomo suprainguinal varicocele repair. Success rates are measured by lack of complication and recurrence. Some series of adolescent varicoceles have looked at testicular catch-up growth as a measure of a successful procedure. A total of 63% to 93% of patients achieved catch up growth postoperatively, which was not affected by ligation of the artery or lymphatics.[59,60] Most series do not include evaluation of semen parameters before or after surgery; however, there is suggestion that artery preservation leads to improved semen analysis results.[54]

CURRENT CONTROVERSIES/FUTURE CONSIDERATIONS

In the treatment of the adolescent patient with a varicocele, information is rarely available regarding the patient's fertility, as the patients are too young. This lack of information hampers the ability to extract meaningful information regarding the efficacy and utility of treatment, whether it is surgical repair or observation. It is therefore important to embark on prospective long-term follow-up studies of these adolescents. A useful proxy to paternity status can be assessed by obtaining semen analyses before and after intervention to evaluate fertility potential.

SUMMARY

- Varicoceles are found in 4% to 15% of adolescents and are commonly asymptomatic.
- Indications for varicocelectomy are left testicular hypotrophy (>10%–20%), abnormal semen analysis, or pain.
- Varicocelectomy can be performed open, laparoscopically, endovascularly, or microscopically.
- The most common complication is a hydrocele; artery- and lymphatic-sparing varicocelectomy diminishes the risk of hydrocele significantly; however, it increases the risk of a residual or recurrent varicocele.
- Critics of the laparoscopic procedure have argued that it does not provide superior outcomes while introducing the significant risks to intra-abdominal contents associated with laparoscopy.

REFERENCES

1. Scorer CG. The descent of the testis. Arch Dis Child 1964;39:605–9.
2. Sijstermans K, Hack WW, Meijer RW, et al. The frequency of undescended testis from birth to adulthood: a review. Int J Androl 2008;31(1):1–11.
3. Thong M, Lim C, Fatimah H. Undescended testes: incidence in 1,002 consecutive male infants and outcome at 1 year of age. Pediatr Surg Int 1998; 13(1):37–41.

4. Wenzler DL, Bloom DA, Park JM. What is the rate of spontaneous testicular descent in infants with cryptorchidism? J Urol 2004;171(2 Pt 1):849–51.

5. Koff SA. Does compensatory testicular enlargement predict monorchism? J Urol 1991;146(2 Pt 2):632–3.

6. Wood HM, Elder JS. Cryptorchidism and testicular cancer: separating fact from fiction. J Urol 2009; 181(2):452–61.

7. Kolon TF, Herndon CD, Baker LA, et al. Evaluation and treatment of cryptorchidism: AUA guideline. J Urol 2014;192(2):337–45.

8. Moller H, Cortes D, Engholm G, et al. Risk of testicular cancer with cryptorchidism and with testicular biopsy: cohort study. BMJ 1998;317(7160):729.

9. Akre O, Pettersson A, Richiardi L. Risk of contralateral testicular cancer among men with unilaterally undescended testis: a meta analysis. Int J Cancer 2009;124(3):687–9.

10. Pettersson A, Richiardi L, Nordenskjold A, et al. Age at surgery for undescended testis and risk of testicular cancer. N Engl J Med 2007;356(18):1835–41.

11. Cobellis G, Noviello C, Nino F, et al. Spermatogenesis and cryptorchidism. Front Endocrinol (Lausanne) 2014;5:63.

12. Cortesi N, Ferrari P, Zambarda E, et al. Diagnosis of bilateral abdominal cryptorchidism by laparoscopy. Endoscopy 1976;8(1):33–4.

13. Caldamone AA, Amaral JF. Laparoscopic stage 2 Fowler-Stephens orchiopexy. J Urol 1994;152(4): 1253–6.

14. Jordan GH, Winslow BH. Laparoscopic single stage and staged orchiopexy. J Urol 1994;152(4):1249–52.

15. Lindgren BW, Darby EC, Faiella L, et al. Laparoscopic orchiopexy: procedure of choice for the nonpalpable testis? J Urol 1998;159(6):2132–5.

16. Daher P, Nabbout P, Feghali J, et al. Is the Fowler-Stephens procedure still indicated for the treatment of nonpalpable intraabdominal testis? J Pediatr Surg 2009;44(10):1999–2003.

17. Elyas R, Guerra LA, Pike J, et al. Is staging beneficial for Fowler-Stephens orchiopexy? A systematic review. J Urol 2010;183(5):2012–8.

18. Emir H, Ayik B, Elicevik M, et al. Histological evaluation of the testicular nubbins in patients with nonpalpable testis: assessment of etiology and surgical approach. Pediatr Surg Int 2007;23(1):41–4.

19. Martin AD, Rushton HG. The prevalence of bell clapper anomaly in the solitary testis in cases of prior perinatal torsion. J Urol 2014;191(Suppl 5): 1573–7.

20. Lorenzo AJ, Samuelson ML, Docimo SG, et al. Cost analysis of laparoscopic versus open orchiopexy in the management of unilateral nonpalpable testicles. J Urol 2004;172(2):712–6.

21. Wein AJ, Kavoussi LR, Campbell MF. Campbell-Walsh urology. 10th edition. In: Wein AJ, Kavoussi LR, Novick AC, et al, editors. Abnormalities of the Testis and Scrotum. Philadelphia: Elsevier Press; 2012. p. 3563–4.

22. Samadi AA, Palmer LS, Franco I. Laparoscopic orchiopexy: report of 203 cases with review of diagnosis, operative technique, and lessons learned. J Endourol 2003;17(6):365–8.

23. Desireddi NV, Liu DB, Maizels M, et al. Magnetic resonance arteriography/venography is not accurate to structure management of the impalpable testis. J Urol 2008;180(Suppl 4):1805–8 [discussion: 1808–9].

24. Tong Q, Zheng L, Tang S, et al. Laparoscopy-assisted orchiopexy for recurrent undescended testes in children. J Pediatr Surg 2009;44(4):806–10.

25. Riquelme M, Aranda A, Rodarte-Shade M, et al. Totally laparoscopic approach for failed conventional orchiopexy. J Laparoendosc Adv Surg Tech A 2012;22(5):514–7.

26. He D, Lin T, Wei G, et al. Laparoscopic orchiopexy for treating inguinal canalicular palpable undescended testis. J Endourol 2008;22(8):1745–9.

27. Riquelme M, Aranda A, Rodriguez C, et al. Laparoscopic orchiopexy for palpable undescended testes: a five-year experience. J Laparoendosc Adv Surg Tech A 2006;16(3):321–4.

28. Baker LA, Docimo SG, Surer I, et al. A multi-institutional analysis of laparoscopic orchiopexy. BJU Int 2001;87(6):484–9.

29. Radmayr C, Oswald J, Schwentner C, et al. Long-term outcome of laparoscopically managed nonpalpable testes. J Urol 2003;170(6 Pt 1):2409–11.

30. Denes FT, Saito FJ, Silva FA, et al. Laparoscopic diagnosis and treatment of nonpalpable testis. Int Braz J Urol 2008;34(3):329–34 [discussion: 335].

31. Esposito C, Garipoli V. The value of 2-step laparoscopic Fowler-Stephens orchiopexy for intra-abdominal testes. J Urol 1997;158(5):1952–4 [discussion: 1954–5].

32. Chang B, Palmer LS, Franco I. Laparoscopic orchiopexy: a review of a large clinical series. BJU Int 2001;87(6):490–3.

33. Dave S, Manaboriboon N, Braga LH, et al. Open versus laparoscopic staged Fowler-Stephens orchiopexy: impact of long loop vas. J Urol 2009; 182(5):2435–9.

34. Yucel S, Ziada A, Harrison C, et al. Decision making during laparoscopic orchiopexy for intra-abdominal testes near the internal ring. J Urol 2007;178(4 Pt 1):1447–50 [discussion: 1450].

35. Handa R, Kale R, Harjai MM. Laparoscopic orchiopexy: is closure of the internal ring necessary? J Postgrad Med 2005;51(4):266–7 [discussion: 268].

36. Hsieh MH, Bayne A, Cisek LJ, et al. Bladder injuries during laparoscopic orchiopexy: incidence and lessons learned. J Urol 2009;182(1):280–4 [discussion: 284–5].

37. Kelalis PP, King LR, Belman AB. Clinical pediatric urology. 2nd edition. Philadelphia: Saunders; 2006.

38. Esposito C, Vallone G, Savanelli A, et al. Long-term outcome of laparoscopic Fowler-Stephens orchiopexy in boys with intra-abdominal testis. J Urol 2009;181(4):1851–6.

39. Esposito C, Vallone G, Settimi A, et al. Laparoscopic orchiopexy without division of the spermatic vessels: can it be considered the procedure of choice in cases of intraabdominal testis? Surg Endosc 2000; 14(7):658–60.

40. Burjonrappa SC, Al Hazmi H, Barrieras D, et al. Laparoscopic orchiopexy: the easy way to go. J Pediatr Surg 2009;44(11):2168–72.

41. Niedzielski J, Paduch D, Raczynski P. Assessment of adolescent varicocele. Pediatr Surg Int 1997; 12(5–6):410–3.

42. Rais A, Zarka S, Derazne E, et al. Varicocoele among 1 300 000 Israeli adolescent males: time trends and association with body mass index. Andrology 2013;1(5):663–9.

43. Zampieri N, Cervellione RM. Varicocele in adolescents: a 6-year longitudinal and followup observational study. J Urol 2008;180(Suppl 4):1653–6 [discussion: 1656].

44. Kolon TF, Clement MR, Cartwright L, et al. Transient asynchronous testicular growth in adolescent males with a varicocele. J Urol 2008;180(3):1111–4 [discussion:1114–5].

45. Poon SA, Gjertson CK, Mercado MA, et al. Testicular asymmetry and adolescent varicoceles managed expectantly. J Urol 2010;183(2):731–4.

46. Preston MA, Carnat T, Flood T, et al. Conservative management of adolescent varicoceles: a retrospective review. Urology 2008;72(1):77–80.

47. Diamond DA, Zurakowski D, Atala A, et al. Is adolescent varicocele a progressive disease process? J Urol 2004;172(4 Pt 2):1746–8 [discussion: 1748].

48. Diegidio P, Jhaveri JK, Ghannam S, et al. Review of current varicocelectomy techniques and their outcomes. BJU Int 2011;108(7):1157–72.

49. Cayan S, Shavakhabov S, Kadioglu A. Treatment of palpable varicocele in infertile men: a meta-analysis to define the best technique. J Androl 2009;30(1):33–40.

50. Borruto FA, Impellizzeri P, Antonuccio P, et al. Laparoscopic vs open varicocelectomy in children and adolescents: review of the recent literature and meta-analysis. J Pediatr Surg 2010;45(12):2464–9.

51. Barroso U Jr, Andrade DM, Novaes H, et al. Surgical treatment of varicocele in children with open and laparoscopic Palomo technique: a systematic review of the literature. J Urol 2009;181(6):2724–8.

52. Chrouser K, Vandersteen D, Crocker J, et al. Nerve injury after laparoscopic varicocelectomy. J Urol 2004;172(2):691–3 [discussion: 693].

53. Muensterer OJ. Genitofemoral nerve injury after laparoscopic varicocelectomy in adolescents. J Urol 2008;180(5):2155–7 [discussion: 2157–8].

54. Zampieri N, Zuin V, Corroppolo M, et al. Varicocele and adolescents: semen quality after 2 different laparoscopic procedures. J Androl 2007;28(5):727–33.

55. Rizkala E, Fishman A, Gitlin J, et al. Long term outcomes of lymphatic sparing laparoscopic varicocelectomy. J Pediatr Urol 2013;9(4):458–63.

56. Lee SW, Lee JY, Kim KH, et al. Laparoendoscopic single-site surgery versus conventional laparoscopic varicocele ligation in men with palpable varicocele: a randomized, clinical study. Surg Endosc 2012;26(4):1056–62.

57. Kang DH, Lee JY, Chung JH, et al. Laparoendoscopic single site varicocele ligation: comparison of testicular artery and lymphatic preservation versus complete testicular vessel ligation. J Urol 2013;189(1):243–9.

58. Bansal D, Riachy E, Defoor WR Jr, et al. Pediatric varicocelectomy: a comparative study of conventional laparoscopic and laparoendoscopic single-site approaches. J Endourol 2014;28(5):513–6.

59. Poon SA, Kozakowski KA, Decastro GJ, et al. Adolescent varicocelectomy: postoperative catch-up growth is not secondary to lymphatic ligation. J Pediatr Urol 2009;5(1):37–41.

60. Kim KS, Lee C, Song SH, et al. Impact of internal spermatic artery preservation during laparoscopic varicocelectomy on recurrence and the catch-up growth rate in adolescents. J Pediatr Urol 2014; 10(3):435–40.

Laparoscopic Nephrectomy and Partial Nephrectomy
Intraperitoneal, Retroperitoneal, Single Site

Paul R. Bowlin, MD, Walid A. Farhat, MD*

KEYWORDS

- Laparoscopy • Nephrectomy • Partial nephrectomy • Retroperitoneal • Single site

KEY POINTS

- Laparoscopy has become a mainstay approach in the management of pediatric renal maladies.
- Transperitoneal and retroperitoneal laparoscopic approaches are safe and effective.
- Advancing technologies, such as single-site surgery and robotics, are becoming increasingly common in the management of pediatric patients.

 Videos of umbilical incision, trocar incision, colon mobilization, transperitoneal nephrectomy, and prone nephrectomy accompany this article at http://www.urologic.theclinics.com/

INTRODUCTION

The indications for simple laparoscopic nephrectomy range from mitigation of renin-mediated hypertension and severe proteinuria, to removal of infected, poorly functioning renal units, or severely hydronephrotic kidneys. The use of minimally invasive surgery (MIS) further extended to malignant pathologies, hence radical laparoscopic nephrectomy is frequently offered for pediatric renal malignancies, such as Wilms tumor or renal cell carcinoma. On the other hand, although partial nephrectomy is traditionally used for management of renal malignancies in adults, its role in the pediatric population is more commonly limited to duplex kidneys with or without ureteroceles.

Historically, laparoscopic nephrectomies in pediatric and infant patients were initially described by Ehrlich and colleagues[1] (pediatric) and Koyle and colleagues[2] (infant) in the early 1990s. In both cases they removed a multicystic dysplastic kidney. Since that time, the general principles of transperitoneal laparoscopic nephrectomy have largely remained the same.

Although pediatric laparoscopy was hindered at first by the size of the access ports and the length of the instrumentation, advances in technology and development of dedicated pediatric instruments have led to fast adoption and dissemination of this surgical approach. Today, there are 3-mm to 5-mm instruments with respective optics widely available, and technical advances by some companies (eg, GIMMI [GIMMI GmbH, Tuttlingen, Germany]; **Fig. 1**) have allowed even further miniaturization to 2.7-mm instruments and optics.

Laparoscopy in children is a unique procedure when compared with adults, and the nuances of this approach in the pediatric population are not only related to size of the patients or instruments, but also pertain to the physiology. For instance, the relative distance between the access point and any intra-abdominal structures has the potential to cause significant damage as instruments are

Disclosures: None.
The Hospital for Sick Children, 555 University Avenue, Toronto, ON M5G 1X8, Canada
* Corresponding author.
E-mail address: walid.farhat@sickkids.ca

Urol Clin N Am 42 (2015) 31–42
http://dx.doi.org/10.1016/j.ucl.2014.09.012

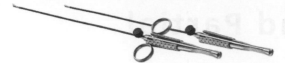

Fig. 1. GIMMI instruments. (*Courtesy of* GIMMI GmbH, Tuttlingen, Germany; with permission.)

advanced into the abdominal or retroperitoneal cavity. In addition, there can be more significant physiologic effects of pneumoperitoneum on the respiratory, cardiovascular, renal, and gastrointestinal tracts, particularly at higher pressures. Surgeons embarking on incorporating laparoscopy in their practice are advised to have a clear and deep understanding of the evolving technology and the physiology of children.

NEPHRECTOMY
Equipment

The array of laparoscopic equipment available in the market today is immense, although still far less so in the pediatric market as compared with the adult market. In general, we prefer to have a standard set up for all laparoscopic renal cases (**Table 1**), with additional specialized equipment available on standby to be used as needed. Standardization of equipment placement and organization of the various cables and tubes is essential for safety and efficiency during the case. For instance, we recommend using a dedicated Mayo stand to keep the basic equipment in a predictable location and easily within reach.

General Positioning

Like any surgical procedure, one of the first, and most critical, steps in a laparoscopic nephrectomy is patient positioning, padding, and retention to the table. We recommend that positioning be done as a joint effort among the surgeon, anesthesiologist, and nursing staff to ensure that all aspects and potential implications of the patient position are accounted for. When performing

simple nephrectomy, positioning can vary from supine to partial flank to full flank, depending on multiple factors, such as body habitus, operative side, kidney size, planned port placement, and anticipated exposure needs. In any of the positions, the break point in the bed and/or kidney rest may be used to help widen the angle between the lower ribs and pelvic brim, effectively increasing the operative space. In general, however, the benefit of the kidney rest and/or bed break is fairly limited in pediatric patients because of their small size. When a partial or full-flank position is used, the positioning of the arms and legs are critical to ensure there is no strain on the respective joints. Once positioning is established, the focus shifts toward appropriately padding pressure points. Once positioned and padded, the patient needs to be secured to the bed with sturdy tape (2–3-inch cloth tape) to provide complete security and allow the bed to be maximally deflected in any direction without risking significant shifting of the patient on the bed. Furthermore, key points that need to be secured with tape include upper and lower legs, hips, chest and shoulders, arms, and head. If simple bed movement is planned, such as mild Trendelenberg, then it is often necessary to tape only the legs and chest/shoulders. Any degree of side-to-side bed adjustment should mandate taping around the hips, arms, and head as well.

TRANSPERITONEAL SIMPLE NEPHRECTOMY
Access

When performing a transabdominal approach, we recommend open access to the peritoneal cavity via the umbilical region, with the point of entry at the fusion of the fascial layers to form the linea alba. We find this anatomic landmark to be the most predictable point of entry into the abdomen.

Once the umbilicus is everted, the lateral aspects are grasped with Allis clamps and skin is incised in a vertical transumbilical fashion using a #11 blade (**Fig. 2**). The open umbilicus is

Table 1
General and specialized laparoscopic equipment

Case	General Equipment	Special Equipment
Nephrectomy or partial nephrectomy	30° scope (3, 5, or 10 mm depending on the procedure to be performed); scissor with cautery, Maryland, bowel, and right-angle graspers; hook; suction irrigator; clip applier; specimen-retrieval bag	Laparoscopic stapler, specialized coagulation device (eg, Harmonic, Enseal, LigaSure, Thunderbeat)
Retroperitoneal nephrectomy or partial nephrectomy		In addition to above, narrow S-retractor or right-angle retractor

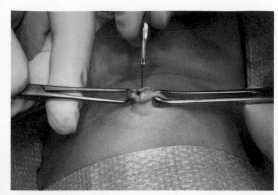

Fig. 2. Umbilical incision for laparoscopic intraperitoneal access.

carefully separated until the point in which the peritoneum joins the skin is seen. Once the peritoneal cavity is entered, the skin is then separated from the peritoneum as described in the Bailez technique (Video 1).[3] A 2-0 absorbable suture u-stitch is placed around the peritoneal opening to facilitate traction during port placement, limit gas leakage around the port, and for use in fascial closure at the conclusion of the case. With the previously placed 2-0 Vicryl in place and before complete tightening of the suture, traction is applied, and the 5-mm or 10-mm laparoscopic trocar is placed. A 30° scope is then inserted under direct vision, and after confirming that the trocar is properly placed intraperitoneally by visualizing, bowels insufflation is started (pressure of 12 mm Hg or less dependent on the age and weight of patient with incremental flow of 1–3 L/min).

Two accessory additional ports are then placed under direct vision. Ideally the 2 working ports are placed along the ipsilateral rectus border. In case splenic or liver retraction is needed, a third accessory port can be placed in the midline just below the xiphoid. Because the abdominal cavity is small and finger pressure may completely obscure and mislead trocar site insertion, we traditionally use the following method. For each port, the target entry site is first identified using a 22-gauge needle while visualized from the intraperitoneal cavity. Once the correct site is adequately identified, local analgesia is injected followed by incision using an 11 blade through the skin, abdominal wall, and peritoneum. Using the same trajectory, a straight hemostat is then used to gently spread the fascia and thereafter the laparoscopic trocar (Video 2). We find that this trocar placement method limits gas leak and decreases the chance of dislodging the trocar, especially in long procedures.

Technical Details

- Mobilization the colon overlying the kidney while maintaining the lateral renal attachments (Video 3).
- Colon is dissected along the white line of Toldt from the splenic flexure on the left or hepatic flexure on the right.
- Once the ureter is identified, as it courses over the psoas muscle, it is followed cephalad to the hilum and can be used for traction.
- The hilum should be carefully dissected using gentle scissor or blunt dissection.
  - The suction irrigator also can be useful as a relatively atraumatic dissection device.
- Efforts should be made to isolate the artery first and vein second.
- Once isolated, the vessels can be ligated separately with clips (**Fig. 3**) and hilum is secured.
- The remaining superior and lateral attachments are divided along with the ureter.
- In certain circumstances and especially when the kidney is hydronephrotic, the hilum may be effaced and is composed of many small vessels that need precise dissection and clipping. Hence, caution should be exercised when dissecting the kidney superiorly or posteriorly to avoid aberrant vessels.

Specimen Removal

With small kidneys being removed for nononcologic indications, the specimen can often be removed via the umbilical incision. The 10-mm lens is exchanged

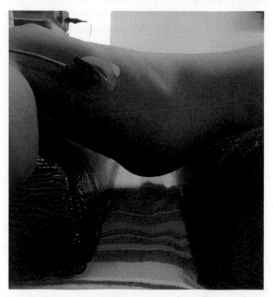

Fig. 3. Prone positioning. Note the ability of the abdomen to expand without compression against the surgical table.

for a 5-mm lens to allow visualization via one of the accessory ports. A 10-mm heavy grasper can be placed through the umbilical port and the specimen removed along with the port. If necessary, the fascial and/or skin incision can be extended to accommodate specimen retrieval. If the specimen is very large or needs to remain intact, such as with a renal tumor, it should be placed in a retrieval bag and extracted via extension of the incision of one of the ports or via an alternate incision, such as a Pfannenstiel incision, in the lower abdomen.

The resection bed should be inspected for hemostasis. Routine placement of a drain is not necessary. Closure of the umbilicus is accomplished at the fascial level by tying down the 2-0 absorbable suture placed during initial access. We do not close the 5-mm port sites and we approximate skin with absorbable suture and skin glue. We consider that the type of trocar (dilating tip) and method we use for trocar insertion to be minimally disruptive to the fascia or overlying muscles hence the risk of hernia is low. In our practice, we have not yet seen any patient presenting with a hernia from the trocar site. Nevertheless, we recommend that surgeons use their own judgment for these minor surgical details.

The key steps of the transperitoneal nephrectomy are shown in Video 4.

Comments

Although transperitoneal laparoscopic nephrectomy is popular, the retroperitoneal approach is considered a neat direct approach to tackle a benign pathology in the pediatric population. Children have minimal perinephric fat and anatomically are very suitable for a retroperitoneal laparoscopic approach.

RETROPERITONEAL FLANK APPROACH

Retroperitoneal laparoscopic nephrectomy in children was first described by Diamond and colleagues[4] in 1995. In this series, patients were positioned in a lateral decubitus position with access established via an incision in the costovertebral angle. Prone positioning also has been used, with access achieved in a similar fashion.[5] Traditionally, enlargement of the retroperitoneal potential space is accomplished using balloon dilators,[6] Foley catheters,[7] condoms,[8] and glove fingers,[9] but we find a soaked wet sponge to be sufficient to create the space in children.

Positioning

When performing a retroperitoneal laparoscopic nephrectomy in the flank position, the patient's back should be flush with the table edge, hence allowing full and free anteroposterior planes for instruments to prevent instrument collision with the surface of the bed when dissecting the renal anterior attachments.

Access

A 1-cm incision is made approximately 1 cm off the tip of the 12th rib. The muscle layers are sequentially split using sharp dissection and advancing the tips the of scissors all the way to the retroperitoneum. Once the tips of the scissors are in the retroperitoneum, narrow right-angle or "S" retractors are used to identify and confirm that the peritoneum is not violated (bowels should not be seen) and retroperitoneal space is reached (presence of perinephric fat, albeit minimal, is seen). A damp sponge is then fed through the incision and into the retroperitoneal space to begin developing the cavity. In children older than 1 year, the entire sponge can generally be inserted. In children younger than 1 year, typically only half of the sponge is needed. With the sponge in place, a 2-0 absorbable suture is placed as a u-stitch on the external fascia to provide traction and minimize gas leak. With traction on the untightened 2-0 Vicryl, a 10-mm trocar is placed into the retroperitoneum, and once perinephric tissues and fat are seen (ie, scope is not in muscle layers), then insufflation initiated. Pressure should be set at 12 mm Hg or less, with flow started at 1 L/min and gradually increased to 3 L/min.

Technical Details

- Dissection and creation of the retroperitoneal space is created with both blunt dissection and the pressure of direct insufflation, using the 30° laparoscope.
- The retroperitoneal space is further developed by moving the camera and trocar as a unit posteriorly along the psoas muscle toward the anterior abdominal wall and then medially to mobilize the peritoneum away from the surgical space.
  - This maneuver needs to be delicate and under vision to avoid violating the peritoneum.
- Once the retroperitoneal space is adequate and edge of peritoneum is medially positioned, the 2 additional 5-mm ports are placed under direct vision.
  - The first port is placed anterior to the paraspinous muscles and traditionally is used to further develop the retroperitoneal space by further mobilizing the peritoneum medially.
  - The second trocar is inserted 10 to 15 mm superior to the anterior superior iliac spine in the axillary line.

○ It is imperative that this anterior port is placed after sufficiently displacing the peritoneum anterior and medially. Failure to do so risks transperitoneal port insertion.

- Once all trocars are in place, the kidney is approached posteriorly so as to identify the renal pedicle.
    ○ A key anatomic landmark is the psoas muscle, which we use to be fully oriented to the retroperitoneal cavity.
- An instrument is typically needed to help lift the kidney away from the psoas muscle to allow visualization and dissection of the renal hilum.
- With the kidney still attached to the peritoneum anteriorly, it is customary to identify the ureter, which makes it quite easy to follow cephalad toward the hilum.
- Ligation of the renal vessels and ureter can be performed.
    ○ The retroperitoneal approach makes it easy to first identify the artery and ligate before visualizing the vein.
    ○ Nevertheless, it is common to again have the vessels effaced by a large hydronephrotic kidney or even small and flattened by a small shrunken renal unit, hence making it easy to miss small vessels, which may cause bleeding if not identified and adequately ligated.

Specimen Removal

As with the transperitoneal approach, the specimen either can be extracted via the larger 10-mm port site (using an alternative port with a 5-mm camera), which often has to be extended, or, if the specimen is larger, removing the kidney in pieces may be achieved. With the intracorporeal space being very small, it is usually difficult to place a retrieval bag.

The 10-mm port site can be closed at the fascial level, with the 2-0 absorbable suture placed during the retroperitoneal access. The remaining port sites are closed at the skin level only with an absorbable suture and skin glue.

Comments

Although the retroperitoneal flank approach provides a direct access to the kidney and hilum, it needs lots of dexterity and may be difficult to teach. For instance, the mere fact that dissection and hilar control may need to be done with one instrument while the other is retracting the kidney anteriorly makes it cumbersome, especially because the space is very limited and may be difficult to accommodate an extra trocar for retraction.

One approach to overcome this surgical limitation is to dissect the whole kidney and then tackle the hilum with the kidney floating in the retroperitoneal space. Although this technique is a useful alternative, it may be difficult to use on all cases, especially when the kidney has aberrant multiple vessels. Thus, we recently incorporated the prone retroperitoneal approach into our surgical armamentarium. This approach is quite permissive, not only because peritoneal cavity violation does not pose any limitation on surgical exposure, but rather because it allows the use of both accessory trocars for dissection and manipulation.

RETROPERITONEAL PRONE APPROACH
Positioning

In the prone approach, the child needs to be positioned between hip and chest pads such that the abdomen is essentially hovering on the surface of the operative table (see **Fig. 3**). This allows the abdominal contents to fall away from the retroperitoneum and, in the event that the peritoneal cavity is inadvertently entered, prevents compression of the retroperitoneum from the resultant pneumoperitoneum.

Access

Retroperitoneal access is achieved via a 1-cm incision at the costovertebral angle, lateral to the sacrospinalis muscle. Blunt dissection is carried down just lateral to the quadratus lumborum muscle to the level of the lumbodorsal fascia. The fascia is a definitive landmark that has resistance but can be bluntly penetrated with the tips of scissors, which signifies entry into the retroperitoneum. As in the flank approach, part or all of a damp sponge is fed through the incision and into the retroperitoneal space to begin developing the cavity. With the sponge in place, a 2-0 absorbable suture is placed as a u-stitch on the fascia. The 10-mm port is placed and insufflation is started. The 30° lens is used along with the pneumoperitoneum to help further delineate the retroperitoneal cavity. Two additional 5-mm ports are placed, one in the posterior midaxillary line approximately 2 cm above the iliac crest, and the other at the tip of the 12th rib. The psoas muscle, which is an important anatomic landmark in traditional retroperitoneal surgery, is anteriorly placed in the prone position; hence, making it difficult to use as a point of reference. To avoid confusion and disorientation, and once we are in the retroperitoneal space we aim toward the Gerota fascia and tend to identify the renal unit with its laterally suspended hilum.

There are numerous other described methods to achieve retroperitoneal access and develop the retroperitoneal space. Choi and colleagues describe use of a Visiport (Covidien) to enter the retroperitoneum. Once properly positioned, the space is developed using insufflation and blunt dissection with the scope.[10] The retroperitoneal space also can be developed using an inflated surgical glove, glove finger, condom, or a dedicated laparoscopic balloon trocar.

Technical Details

- Dissection and specimen extraction are carried out in the same manner as described with the flank approach although with the prone approach.
- There is no need to lift the kidney away from the psoas muscle, as it will naturally fall away due to gravity; this is one of the unique advantages of the prone approach.
- The hilar vessels are approached in the same manner as in the flank retroperitoneal approach.
- Herein the vessels can be easily ligated and tied rather than only clipped, because the 2 accessory trocars are freely used.
- Closure is also similar to the flank approach, with the 10-mm port site fascia being closed using the initial 2-0 absorbable suture and remaining port sites being closed with absorbable suture and skin glue.

The key steps of the retroperitoneal nephrectomy are shown in Video 5.

COMPARISON OF TRANSPERITONEAL AND RETROPERITONEAL APPROACHES

Several studies have been performed to compare outcomes between transperitoneal and retroperitoneal nephrectomy. Recently, Kim and colleagues[11] performed a systematic review revealing no significant advantage of a retroperitoneal versus transperitoneal approach. There are, however, instances in which one approach is more favorable than another. For instance, in children with multiple previous transabdominal operations, a retroperitoneal approach can be advantageous, as it avoids having to address prior adhesions and scars. Similarly, in children with end-stage renal disease on peritoneal dialysis, it is preferable to avoid the peritoneal cavity so as to not compromise the ability to use the peritoneal dialysis catheter.

Nevertheless, the best approach is determined by multiple factors, including pathology, patient comorbidities, prior abdominal operations, and surgeon comfort. In the relatively straightforward patient without prior abdominal surgery, the transperitoneal approach provides familiar and reliable access to the kidney. In patients with multiple prior abdominal operations or peritoneal dialysis catheters, we favor the prone approach, as it avoids dissection within the peritoneal cavity and takes advantage of gravity to help dissect the kidney posteriorly and identify the hilum.

PARTIAL NEPHRECTOMY
Access

The access techniques for laparoscopic transperitoneal and retroperitoneal (flank or prone) partial nephrectomy are identical to those used in simple/radical laparoscopic nephrectomies. The earliest reports used a transperitoneal approach,[12] but retroperitoneal approaches also have been described.[13] In pediatric patients, the most common pathology requiring partial nephrectomy is nonfunctioning moiety in a duplex system. Although the goal is usually to remove the nonfunctioning moiety, it is mandatory to state that the primary objective of this procedure is to preserve the functioning moiety.

Technical Details

- Although not always necessary, identification of the correct moiety and associated ureter can be facilitated by performing initial cystoscopy and ureteral stent placement in the healthy lower pole ureter.
- After mobilizing the colon medially, the stented ureter and dilated ureter will be easily seen.
- When the dilated nonstented upper pole ureter is identified, we suggest dissecting it off the healthy ureter close to the lower pole of the kidney.
- Once fully isolated from the lower pole ureter, tie or clip it proximally and transect distally.
  - Do not focus or give attention to the distal part (this can be completed after completion of the upper pole heminephrectomy).
- The tie or clip is very helpful in keeping the nonfunctioning moiety dilated.
- Use the proximal clipped ureter as a handle and lift it up periodically toward the abdominal wall.
  - This will provide an indication of the hilum (stretched) and help identify where the ureter is passing under the hilum.
- Once the proximal upper pole ureter is dissected off the hilum inferiorly, the ureter can be passed from under the hilum superiorly.
- The upper pole vessels are usually small and intimate to the ureter. They are commonly effaced (flat) and distinct from the main hilar vessels.

- They do not need more than just a clip or specialized cautery/ligation device.
- With the retroperitoneal approach, particularly when prone, this dissection is often easier with gravity-assisted retraction of the kidney away from the hilum.
- Even before ligation of the vessels, it is possible to see a demarcation line between the functioning and nonfunctioning poles, which can be cut with any type of electrosurgical device.

Upper Pole Heminephrectomy

The upper and lower pole vessels are identified and the upper pole vessels selectively ligated. Use of the Maryland and right-angle graspers is recommended to help facilitate this atraumatic dissection. With the retroperitoneal approach, particularly when prone, this dissection is often easier given the limited dissection needed to identify the renal hilum and the natural gravity-assisted retraction of the kidney away from the hilum. Once ligated, the ischemic upper pole can be seen by the color demarcation relative to the lower pole. The peritoneal attachments to the upper pole should be incised before dividing the parenchyma. The parenchyma can then be divided with a ligating device, such as the Harmonic or Enseal scissor (Ethicon Cincinnati, OH, USA), LigaSure (Covidien, Mansfield, MA, USA), Thunderbeat (Olympus, Center Valley, PA, USA), or just with simple electrocautery scissors. If the upper pole vessels cannot be identified, the upper pole dissection can still be performed carefully with efforts to identify any upper pole vessels, as the dissection proceeds medially. If the upper pole is associated with a nonrefluxing ureter, the distal ureteral stump is left open. If it is a refluxing system, the upper pole ureteral dissection is carried caudally as far as possible and ligated with a clip or suture.

Lower Pole Heminephrectomy

In the case of a lower pole partial nephrectomy, the vessels need to be fully isolated before incising the renal parenchyma. Lower pole mobilization should be minimized so as to avoid inadvertent damage to the renal pedicle. As with the upper pole, the use of blunt graspers is recommended to minimize trauma and facilitate definitive identification of the appropriate polar vessels. Once the vessels and parenchyma are fully dissected and divided, the lower pole ureter is mobilized to near the bladder and ligated to minimize urine reflux into the ureteral stump.

Comments

There are numerous other partial nephrectomy techniques described in the literature. Piaggio and colleagues described a transperitoneal technique, which begins with mobilization of the ureter so it can be used for suprahilar retraction. This is followed by division of the parenchyma and distal ureteral mobilization and ligation.[14] This technique avoids initial dissection around the renal hilum, which helps reduce the risk of compromise to the healthy remaining renal moiety.

As with total nephrectomy, comparison of outcomes from trans versus retroperitoneal partial nephrectomy has not yielded any significant differences.[15] In our experience, however, we find that retroperitoneal heminephrectomy is quite demanding, especially in the very young age group. The potential space of the retroperitoneum is far less than that of the intraperitoneal cavity and often cannot accommodate the spaced needed to adequately dissect and safely identify the renal moiety being removed. Careful preoperative assessment of the patient's size is imperative if considering a retroperitoneal approach. Laparoscopic partial nephrectomy for pediatric malignancy is rarely described in the literature, although Rauth and colleagues[16] described a case accomplished via a transperitoneal approach. In this case, hilar control/occlusion was not required and the specimen was excised using an electrosurgical device.

COMPLICATIONS

With any minimally invasive kidney operation, it is critical to understand how to anticipate and recognize intraoperative complications as well as how to deal with complications as they occur. Understandably, complications may occur from the time the patient gets on the operating table until discharge time, but here we focus on intraoperative complications. The potential for surgical complications begins with patient positioning. Nerve injuries, pressure injuries, and abrasions can all occur as a result of improper positioning. During intraperitoneal access, vascular and bowel injuries can occur, along with the risk of gas embolism. During dissection, one can injure adjacent organs, such as the liver, spleen, pancreas, bowel, and diaphragm. Major vascular injury, both at the hilum and involving adjacent vasculature, is one of the most acutely worrisome events and can necessitate conversion to an open procedure to safely address. Complications, common etiologies, and management are listed in **Table 2**.

Table 2
Laparoscopic complications, etiology, and management

Complication	Frequent Etiology	Management
Gas embolism	Unrecognized venous injury or penetration	Release of pneumoperitoneum, reposition patient left side down/head down, assess need for additional intervention with anesthesia
Bowel injury	Initial peritoneal access, instrument trauma, thermal, perirenal dissection	Primary closure (laparoscopic or open), bowel resection and/or diversion if severely injured
Vascular injury (nonrenal)	Initial peritoneal access, instrument trauma, thermal	Immediate pressure/clamping, assess for ability to manage laparoscopically vs conversion to open
Renal hilum injury	Hilar dissection, excessive traction	Immediate pressure/clamping, assess for ability to manage laparoscopically vs conversion to open
Vascular injury (renal)	Damage to accessory renal vessel, adrenal artery or vein	Immediate pressure/clamping, assess for ability to manage laparoscopically vs conversion to open
Pancreatic injury	Dissection near upper pole of kidney	Consultation with general surgeon to assist with management
Splenic injury	Dissection around upper pole of left kidney	Minor injury: focal cautery and/or compression and/or hemostatic agent Major injury: consultation with general surgeon to assist with management
Liver injury	Dissection around upper pole of right kidney	Minor injury: focal cautery and/or compression and/or hemostatic agent Major injury: consultation with general surgeon to assist with management
Diaphragmatic injury	Lateral dissection around kidney	Minor injury: prompt closure with evacuation of pneumothorax Major injury: consultation with general surgeon to assist with management
Epigastric vessel injury	Port placement	Placement of u-stitch proximal and distal to injury
Renal parenchymal bleeding	Renal dissection, inability to control following partial nephrectomy	Focal cautery, suture ligation, hemostatic agent, packing/compression
Hematoma	Incomplete vascular control	Stable: conservative management (observation) Unstable: radiologic embolization vs surgical exploration
Urinoma	Unrecognized entry into collecting system	Asymptomatic: observation Symptomatic (eg, ileus, fever): ureteral stent and/or percutaneous drain placement
Ischemia	Renal hilar damage, accessory vessel damage, renal torsion	Acute: radiologic vs surgical revascularization Late: observation
Nerve injury	Inadequate padding or improper positioning	Transient: observation, physical therapy Chronic: referral to neurologist

One of the unique, and most feared, complications of partial nephrectomy is damage to, or loss of, the remaining renal moiety. In retroperitoneal cases, stretch injury, especially in the flank position when the kidney needs to be lifted anteriorly, may cause spasm and vascular injury, especially in young children. Vascular injuries or inadvertent ligation of a vessel to the normal renal moiety are the most common etiologies and reinforce the importance of meticulous dissection and careful identification of all vessels before ligation. Damage to the remaining ureter or renal pelvis can lead to ureteral stricture or urine leak. In addition, cystic lesions can be seen in place of the excised renal moiety, as shown in **Fig. 4**.

ADVANCED TECHNOLOGIES

As the collective skill with laparoscopic surgery across all techniques has increased, efforts have been made to develop technologies that allow completion of the procedure with smaller instruments, better dexterity, and enhanced cosmesis. Single-port devices, smaller instrumentation, and robotic surgery systems have all contributed to these goals.

SINGLE PORT

One of the initial "single-port" laparoscopic articles described a technique to mobilize the appendix (with extracorporeal ligation) in pediatric patients.[17] Early reports of multi-instrument single-port laparoscopic nephrectomy were in the adult literature.[18] Its use in pediatric nephrectomy was first described in 2009 by Johnson and colleagues.[19] The emergence of new and updated technology related to port design, instrument design, and optics has allowed greater integration of the technology. In 2010, Koh and colleagues[20] described their early experience with single-site surgery for pediatric nephrectomy in 11 patients. To date, single-port laparoscopy has been described for simple, radical, and partial nephrectomies via transperitoneal and retroperitoneal approaches. An overview of several of our preferred single-port systems, instruments, and optics is summarized in **Table 3**. In addition, there are techniques described that use port placement through a surgical glove that is secured to a single-port–type incision.[3,21]

Technical Details

- Placement of any of the single-port systems for transperitoneal nephrectomy or partial nephrectomy can be anywhere on the abdomen.
  - Typically the most optimal cosmetic outcome is achieved via an umbilical incision.
- The size of the skin and fascial incisions vary depending on the particular single-port technology being used.
  - In all cases, and although skin incision may be concealed with the inverted umbilicus, a generous fascial incision is usually needed for the single-port instrument to be adequately placed.
- A 2-cm to 3-cm infraumbilical incision is made and carried down to the fascia.
- A vertical incision is made in the fascia and the peritoneal cavity inspected with a finger for any significant adhesions.
- Placement of the port varies depending on the technology.
  - In general, although the port is placed inside the peritoneal cavity, it is then held in place against the abdominal wall by a retaining ring, flange, or screw thread.
  - Care should be given to the possibility of bowel entrapment between the laparo-endoscopic single-site surgery instrument and abdominal wall, hence finger and later visual inspection should be routinely performed.
- Pneumoperitoneum is established and dissection is accomplished by using techniques and concepts derived from traditional laparoscopy.

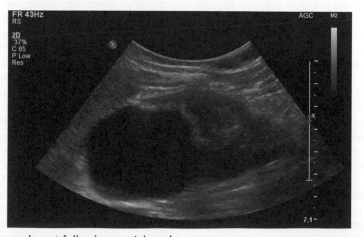

Fig. 4. Residual upper pole cyst following partial nephrectomy.

Table 3
Examples of some of our preferred single-port technologies

Manufacturer	Device Name	Disposable
Advanced Surgical Concepts/ Olympus	QuadPort	Yes
	TriPort	Yes
	TriPort 15	Yes
	ENDOEYE	No
	HiQ LS	No
Applied Medical	GelPOINT	Yes
	GelPOINT Mini	Yes
	Epix	Yes
Covidien	SILS Port	Yes
	SILS Hand Instruments	Yes
	SILS Stitch	Yes
Karl Storz	ENDOCONE	No
	XCONE	No
	DAPRI	No

Advanced Surgical Concepts (Bray, Co Wicklow, Ireland), Olympus (Center Valley, PA, USA), Applied Medical (Rancho Santa, Margarita, CA, USA), Covidien (Mansfield, MA, USA), Karl Storz (Tuttlingen, Germany).

Specimen Removal

Once the specimen is ready for removal, it can be withdrawn directly through the port site or placed in a retrieval bag with extraction via the port site. If the specimen is too large to fit through the port site, the incision can be extended or the specimen can be removed via an alternate site. The latter option, however, begins to negate the cosmetic advantage of a single-port operation.

Comments

The challenge of any single-port operation is not in the anatomic dissection, as these steps are familiar to anyone who has performed traditional laparoscopy, but in the physical ability to perform the various dissecting, ligating, and excising maneuvers given the limited range of motion and fixed fulcrum point associated with the single port. Techniques to address these challenges include use of prebent or deflectable instruments, offset optics, altered instrument positioning (such as holding an instrument upside down to limit handpiece collision), or using instruments/scopes of different lengths. Although traditional laparoscopic instruments have been used, many advantages are gained by the use of specialized single-port instrumentation. The number and variety of single-port systems, instruments, and imaging technology has advanced rapidly. Instruments fall in to 3 main categories: straight, prebent, and articulating (see **Table 3**). Variations in hand-piece and working element design also facilitate efficient use. Optic technology now includes access to deflectable cameras, which help to alleviate external device collision and also provide visual perspective within the peritoneal cavity. In addition, the development of 3-dimensional camera systems has provided another option to help enhance the operation.

Although there is no consensus on the duration of the learning curve or optimum method for determining proficiency in single-port surgery, it is reasonable to assume that even experienced laparoscopic surgeons will require significant time to achieve the success that has been demonstrated with traditional laparoscopy. Complex dissections and tasks, such as intracorporeal suturing/knot tying, are particularly challenging to master given the limited working space and ergonomics of single-port surgery. Regardless, single-port surgery has been shown to be feasible and capable of achieving equivalent outcomes to traditional laparoscopy. As the various technologies mature, and new technologies emerge, it will likely become increasingly used in the management of pediatric patients.

ROBOTIC SURGICAL SYSTEMS

The advent of robotic surgical systems has effectively provided another means by which a surgeon can perform any of the aforementioned laparoscopic operations. Theoretic advantages of the robotic approach include enhanced visualization, correction of tremor, improved surgeon ergonomics, and greater range of motion by way of wristed instruments. Disadvantages include cost and instrument size with most the robotic instruments requiring 8-mm ports. Although 5-mm instrument technology has been developed, it currently lacks the same degree of intraperitoneal mobility given limitations in wrist articulation. Currently, Intuitive Surgical is the primary company (Sunnyvale, CA, USA) producing robotic surgical systems. Although there are subtle differences in access and port placement, the main steps of the operation mimic those used in laparoscopy. The robotic platform has been used in pediatrics: simple nephrectomy, radical nephrectomy, and partial nephrectomy for benign indications,[4,22] as well as oncologic.[5,23]

Recently, Gargollo reported a novel technique using robotic-assisted laparoscopy called hidden incision endoscopic surgery.[24] In this technique, the working port incisions are placed along a Pfannenstiel incision line along with a single peri-umbilical port. In his series of 12 patients, which included 2 nephroureterectomies, he demonstrated an enhanced cosmetic result with scars visible only along the normally hidden Pfannenstiel line and in the peri-umbilical region.

Although robotic surgery can provide an enhanced approach to traditional laparoscopic or single-port operations, the current cost and instrument size factors limit its applicability for pediatric patients. Of all the issues, cost is one of the most significant factors that needs to be considered. Although the cost of traditional laparoscopy versus robotic-assisted nephrectomy has not been directly compared, data from the pyeloplasty literature show a relatively similar cost between open and laparoscopic approaches and a significant increase in cost with a robotic approach.[7,25] A recent article by Bansal and colleagues[26] compared single-site laparoscopic nephroureterectomy costs to those of a robotic-assisted operation and noted a 30% increase in cost with a robotic-assisted approach.[8] Although it is reasonable to consider a robotic-assisted operation in complex nephron-sparing operations, in our opinion, the most reasonable option for straightforward nephrectomy and partial nephrectomy continues to be traditional or single-port laparoscopy.

SUMMARY

Laparoscopy has become a fundamental part of any pediatric urologist's surgical repertoire. Advances in techniques and technology have eased some of the initial limitations posed by a laparoscopic approach. Transperitoneal and retroperitoneal (flank or prone) approaches provide reliable access to the kidney and can be selectively used based on the surgical indication. Single-port technology is a more recent advance that will likely continue to gain momentum as a mainstay of pediatric laparoscopy. Robotic surgery is gaining in popularity and availability for many of the operations traditionally done laparoscopically. Only time will determine its overall utility in pediatric renal surgery.

The development of laparoscopic competency related to patient selection, technical skills, and management of postoperative issues is now a core element to surgeon education. The maintenance and maturation of this knowledge is paramount, as these techniques will remain critical to the management of pediatric patients for the foreseeable future.

SUPPLEMENTARY DATA

Supplementary data related to this article can be found online at http://dx.doi.org/10.1016/j.ucl. 2014.09.012.

REFERENCES

1. Ehrlich RM, Gershman A, Mee S, et al. Laparoscopic nephrectomy in a child: expanding horizons for laparoscopy in pediatric urology. J Endourol 1992;6(6): 463–5.
2. Koyle MA, Woo HH, Kavoussi LR. Laparoscopic nephrectomy in the first year of life. J Pediatr Surg 1993;28(5):693–5. Available at: http://eutils.ncbi.nlm. nih.gov/entrez/eutils/elink.fcgi?dbfrom=pubmed&id= 8340861&retmode=ref&cmd=prlinks.
3. Franc-Guimond J, Kryger J, González R. Experience with the Bailez technique for laparoscopic access in children. J Urol 2003;170(3):936–8. http://dx.doi.org/ 10.1097/01.ju.0000081639.66752.e4.
4. Diamond DA, Price HM, McDougall EM, et al. Retroperitoneal laparoscopic nephrectomy in children. J Urol 1995;153(6):1966–8.
5. Borer JG, Cisek LJ, Atala A, et al. Pediatric retroperitoneoscopic nephrectomy using 2 mm. instrumentation. J Urol 1999;162(5):1725–9 [discussion: 1730].
6. Gaur DD. Laparoscopic operative retroperitoneoscopy: use of a new device. J Urol 1992;148(4): 1137–9.
7. Shah A, Chandran H. Use of Foley's catheter to gain access for retroperitoneoscopy. ANZ J Surg 2004; 74(11):1015. http://dx.doi.org/10.1111/j.1445-1433. 2004.03222.x.
8. Gaur DD, Agarwal DK, Purohit KC, et al. Laparoscopic condom dissection: new technique of retroperitoneoscopy. J Endourol 1994;8(2):149–51.
9. Keizur JJ, Tashima M, Das S. Retroperitoneal laparoscopic renal biopsy. Surg Laparosc Endosc 1993; 3(1):60–2.
10. Choi JM, Bayne AP, Bian SX, et al. A single-center experience with prone retroperitoneoscopic versus open renal surgery in children: an age- and procedure-matched comparison. J Endourol 2011;25(9):1563–72. http://dx.doi.org/10.1089/end.2010.0699.
11. Kim C, McKay K, Docimo SG. Laparoscopic nephrectomy in children: systematic review of transperitoneal and retroperitoneal approaches. Urology 2009;73(2):280–4. http://dx.doi.org/10. 1016/j.urology.2008.08.471.
12. Jordan GH, Winslow BH. Laparoendoscopic upper pole partial nephrectomy with ureterectomy. J Urol 1993;150(3):940–3.
13. El-Ghoneimi A, Valla JS, Steyaert H, et al. Laparoscopic renal surgery via a retroperitoneal approach in children. J Urol 1998;160(3 Pt 2):1138–41.
14. Piaggio L, Franc-Guimond J, Figueroa TE, et al. Comparison of laparoscopic and open partial nephrectomy for duplication anomalies in children. J Urol 2006;175(6):2269–73. http://dx.doi.org/10. 1016/S0022-5347(06)00342-9.
15. Smaldone MC, Polsky E, Ricchiuti DJ, et al. Advances in pediatric urologic laparoscopy.

ScientificWorldJournal 2007;7:727–41. http://dx.doi.org/10.1100/tsw.2007.141.

16. Rauth TP, Slone J, Crane G, et al. Laparoscopic nephron-sparing resection of synchronous Wilms tumors in a case of hyperplastic perilobar nephroblastomatosis. J Pediatr Surg 2011;46(5):983–8. http://dx.doi.org/10.1016/j.jpedsurg.2011.01.025.

17. Esposito C. One-trocar appendectomy in pediatric surgery. Surg Endosc 1998;12(2):177–8.

18. Kaouk JH, Haber GP, Goel RK, et al. Single-port laparoscopic surgery in urology: initial experience. Urology 2008;71(1):3–6. http://dx.doi.org/10.1016/j.urology.2007.11.034.

19. Johnson KC, Cha DY, DaJusta DG, et al. Pediatric single-port-access nephrectomy for a multicystic, dysplastic kidney. J Pediatr Urol 2009;5(5):402–4. http://dx.doi.org/10.1016/j.jpurol.2009.03.011.

20. Koh CJ, De Filippo RE, Chang AY, et al. Laparoendoscopic single-site nephrectomy in pediatric patients: initial clinical series of infants to adolescents. Urology 2010;76(6):1457–61. http://dx.doi.org/10.1016/j.urology.2010.06.066.

21. Hong TH, Kim HL, Lee YS, et al. Transumbilical single-port laparoscopic appendectomy (TUSPLA): scarless intracorporeal appendectomy. J Laparoendosc Adv Surg Tech A 2009;19(1):75–8. http://dx.doi.org/10.1089/lap.2008.0338.

22. Mason MD, Anthony Herndon CD, Smith-Harrison LI, et al. Robotic-assisted partial nephrectomy in duplicated collecting systems in the pediatric population: techniques and outcomes. J Pediatr Urol 2014;10(2):374–9. http://dx.doi.org/10.1016/j.jpurol.2013.10.014.

23. Cost NG, Geller JI, Defoor WR, et al. A robotic-assisted laparoscopic approach for pediatric renal cell carcinoma allows for both nephron-sparing surgery and extended lymph node dissection. J Pediatr Surg 2012;47(10):1946–50. http://dx.doi.org/10.1016/j.jpedsurg.2012.08.017.

24. Gargollo PC. Hidden incision endoscopic surgery: description of technique, parental satisfaction and applications. J Urol 2011;185(4):1425–31. http://dx.doi.org/10.1016/j.juro.2010.11.054.

25. Varda BK, Johnson EK, Clark C, et al. National trends of perioperative outcomes and costs for open, laparoscopic and robotic pediatric pyeloplasty. J Urol 2014;191(4):1090–5. http://dx.doi.org/10.1016/j.juro.2013.10.077.

26. Bansal D, Cost NG, Bean CM, et al. Comparison of pediatric robotic-assisted laparoscopic nephroureterectomy and laparoendoscopic single-site nephroureterectomy. Urology 2014;83(2):438–42. http://dx.doi.org/10.1016/j.urology.2013.08.066.

The Laparoscopic Pyeloplasty
Is There a Role in the Age of Robotics?

Mallikarjun N. Reddy, MS, MCh, Rajendra B. Nerli, MS, MCh*

KEYWORDS

- Minimally invasive surgery • Laparoscopy • Pediatrics • Robotic surgery • Da Vinci surgery
- Ureteropelvic junction obstruction

KEY POINTS

- Ureteropelvic junction (UPJ) obstruction is a common anomaly, and presents clinically in all pediatric age groups.
- The past 3 decades have witnessed an evolution in the surgical correction of UPJ obstruction on several fronts, with open surgical techniques yielding way to endoscopic, laparoscopic, and robotic-assisted approaches.
- Robotic-assisted surgery has several advantages in complex laparoscopic reconstructive procedures such as pyeloplasty.
- Comparative studies of laparoscopic and robot-assisted repairs have demonstrated similar success rates.
- Laparoscopic pyeloplasty is here to stay because of its advantages of safety, efficacy, decreased morbidity, reduced hospital stay, and, perhaps most importantly, cost-effectiveness.

INTRODUCTION

Ureteropelvic junction (UPJ) obstruction is a common anomaly, and presents clinically in all pediatric age groups (**Figs. 1** and **2**). There tends to be a clustering in the neonatal period because of the detection of antenatal hydronephrosis, and again later in life because of symptomatic occurrence. Today most cases are identified and diagnosed in the perinatal period.[1]

The past 3 decades have witnessed an evolution in the surgical correction of UPJ obstruction on several fronts, with open surgical techniques yielding way to endoscopic, laparoscopic, and robotic-assisted approaches. Among the various open surgical techniques, the Anderson-Hynes pyeloplasty has become the most commonly used open surgical procedure for the repair of UPJ.[2] The principal reasons for the universal acceptance of the Anderson-Hynes dismembered pyeloplasty have been (1) broad applicability, including preservation of lower pole or crossing vessels, (2) excision of the pathologic UPJ with appropriate repositioning, and (3) successful reduction pyeloplasty. This operation is generally easy to perform and can be accomplished by several surgical approaches, including anterior subcostal, flank, and posterior lumbotomy.[2] Recent advances in equipment and surgical techniques have made minimally invasive surgery (MIS) a well-tolerated and efficient option in the management of UPJ obstruction.

Division of Pediatric Urology, Department of Urology, KLES Kidney Foundation, KLES Dr Prabhakar Kore Hospital and MRC, KLES University's JN Medical College, Belgaum 590010, India
* Corresponding author.
E-mail addresses: director@kleskf.org; rajendranerli@yahoo.in

Urol Clin N Am 42 (2015) 43–52
http://dx.doi.org/10.1016/j.ucl.2014.09.004
0094-0143/15/$ – see front matter © 2015 Elsevier Inc. All rights reserved.

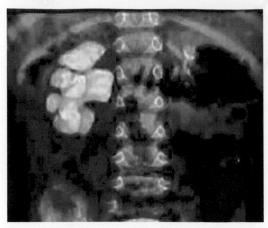

Fig. 1. Intravenous urogram showing right ureteropelvic junction (UPJ) obstruction in a 2-month-old child.

LAPAROSCOPIC PYELOPLASTY
History

Laparoscopic pyeloplasty was first reported in the adult population in 1993 by Kavoussi and Peters[3] and Schuessler and colleagues.[4] Tan[5] reported the first pediatric series of transperitoneal laparoscopic dismembered pyeloplasty in 18 children aged 3 months to 15 years. Yeung and colleagues[6] described their initial experience with laparoscopic retroperitoneal dismembered pyeloplasty

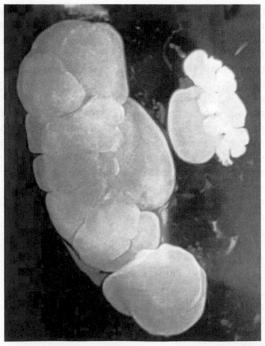

Fig. 2. Magnetic resonance urogram showing bilateral UPJ obstruction in an infant.

in 13 children, 1 of whom required open conversion. El Ghoneimi and colleagues[7] reported their experience of 50 retroperitoneal laparoscopic pyeloplasties in children aged 22 months to 15 years. Similarly, Reddy and colleagues[8] performed laparoscopic pyeloplasties in 16 children, 5 months to 11 years old. During the early 2000s many such small series reported the feasibility of laparoscopic pyeloplasty in children.

Technique

Transperitoneal access
An enema is administered the night before surgery to ensure that the colon is empty. Intraoperative antibiotics are administered to minimize the risk of infection. Patients are catheterized before surgery and the catheter left on free drainage during the operation. Patients are positioned in the lateral position and secured by placing a sand bag to support the back. Patients are further stabilized by strapping the iliac crest to the operating table with an adhesive bandage. Patients are placed as close as possible to the edge of the operating table. The first port is created by open laparoscopy using a blunt Hasson cannula through the umbilical skin crease. A purse-string suture is secured tightly around the Hasson trocar. The abdomen is insufflated with CO_2 to 10 to 12 mm Hg. A single 5-mm instrument port and a single 3-mm instrument port are required. Correct placement of these ports is critical to the ease of performing the anastomosis. Occasionally an extra 5-mm port is placed for retraction purposes. The peritoneum overlying the exposed kidney is incised just lateral to and above the colonic flexure. The loose adventitia around the kidney is detached from the renal capsule. Once the correct plane is identified, the renal capsule is traced into the renal sinus until the renal pelvis is identified. The renal pelvis is further dissected free from the medial side. The UPJ and proximal ureter are identified (**Fig. 3**A). The adventitia around the proximal ureter and UPJ is cleared. The ureter is dismembered with a small cuff of renal pelvis, leaving a 1.5- to 2.0-cm pyelotomy to reanastomose to the ureter (see **Fig. 3**C). The lateral wall of the ureter is opened longitudinally and spatulated (see **Fig. 3**D) for about 1.5 to 2.0 cm along its lateral margin. The UPJ and proximal ureter attached at this point to the spatulated ureter are then excised. The ureteropelvic anastomosis is performed with an 18-cm 6-0 polyglactin suture on a three-eighths round-bodied needle. The first suture is placed at the apex of the spatulated ureter from outside in, then driven through the most dependent part of the pyelotomy. The posterior

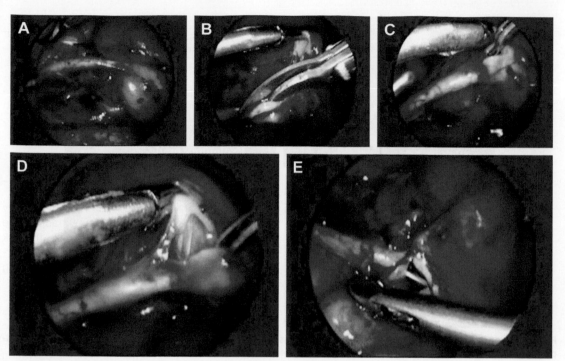

Fig. 3. Transperitoneal laparoscopic pyeloplasty. (*A*) UPJ dissected. (*B*) Pyelotomy done. (*C*) Extension of pyelotomy. (*D*) Pyelotomy incision being carried further down to spatulate the ureter. (*E*) Ureteropelvic anastomosis.

anastomosis is completed running up the length of the spatulated ureter and pelvis. A 0.025-inch guide wire is then passed through the proximal ureter into the bladder. A 3F multilength double-pigtail catheter is passed over the guide wire into the bladder. Next, the proximal end of the double-pigtail stent is placed within the renal pelvis. The anterior anastomosis is then completed as a continuous layer (see **Fig. 3**E). Postoperatively, the drain is removed when less than 5 mL per 24 hours is draining. The catheter is removed the next day. Oral fluids and feeding are started at the appearance of peristaltic sounds. Children are followed for urinary tract infection, and renography is repeated at 3 months.

Retroperitoneal approach

The child is positioned in a lateral or semilateral decubitus position, and 3 to 4 laparoscopic ports are inserted at the surgeon's discretion. Retroperitoneal access is achieved through the first trocar incision 15 mm long and 10 mm from the lower border of the tip of the 12th rib. The Gerota fascia is approached by a muscle-splitting blunt dissection, then opened under direct vision. An index finger is introduced to push the peritoneum forward, thus creating a retroperitoneal cavity. A modification of Gaur balloon technique is used to dissect the retroperitoneum. Two index fingers of

a powder-free surgical glove are placed, one inside the other and ligated onto the 5/10-mm trocar sheath. The dissection is then performed by instilling 500 mL of warm saline through the insufflation channel of the trocar. After completed dissection, the trocar is reinserted without the balloon and pneumoperitoneum established (maximum pressure 12 mm Hg). The first trocar is fixed with a purse-string suture applied around the deep fascia, to ensure an airtight seal. A 5/10-mm telescope is inserted through the first trocar. A second 3/5-mm trocar is inserted posteriorly near the costovertebral angle, while the third 3/5-mm trocar is inserted 1 cm above the top of the iliac crest at the anterior axillary line. To avoid transperitoneal insertion of this trocar, the working space is fully developed and the deep surface of the anterior wall muscles identified before the trocar is inserted. The insufflation pressure is maintained at less than 12 mm Hg and the flow rate of CO_2 is progressively increased from 1 to 3 L/min. The Gerota fascia is incised parallel to the psoas muscle and the perirenal fat is dissected to reveal the lower pole of the kidney, which is then mobilized. The UPJ is identified (**Fig. 4**A) and minimal dissection is used to free the UPJ from connective tissue; small vessels are divided after bipolar electrocoagulation. If needed, a fourth 3/5-mm trocar is inserted lateral to the lumbosacral muscles near

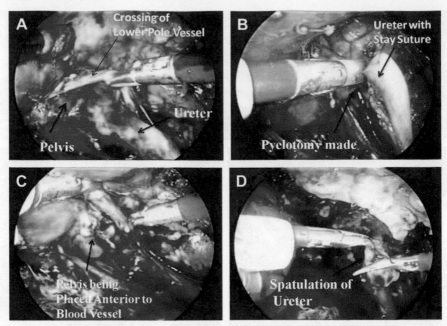

Fig. 4. Retroperitoneal laparoscopic pyeloplasty. (*A*) Dissection of UPJ, crossing vessel lifted from UPJ. (*B*) Pyelotomy made. (*C*) Pelvis is placed anterior to crossing lower pole vessel. (*D*) Ureter is spatulated.

the iliac crest. A stay suture of 5-0 absorbable suture material is placed at the UPJ for traction. The anterior surface of the UPJ is cleared to identify any crossing vessels. The renal pelvis (see **Fig. 4**B) is partly divided by scissors at the most dependent part, while light traction on the stay suture is helpful for manipulating the UPJ maintaining under mild traction. The ureter is partly divided and incised vertically for spatulation (see **Fig. 4**D). The traction suture helps to mobilize the ureter so that the scissors can be in the axis of the ureter. The anterior surface of the kidney is left adherent to the peritoneum so that the kidney is retracted medially with no need for individual kidney retraction. The pelviureteric anastomosis (**Fig. 5**A) begins using 6-0 absorbable sutures and a tapered 3/8 circular needle. The first suture is placed from the most dependent portion of the pelvis to the most inferior point or vertex of the ureteric spatulation. The suture is tied using the intracorporeal technique with the knots placed outside the lumen. The same suture is used on the anterior wall of the anastomosis. The UPJ is maintained on traction and the suture line stabilized. A 4.5F polyurethrane double-J stent (see **Fig. 5**B) is inserted through the suture line to the bladder at the end of the anterior layer reconstruction (see **Fig. 5**C). The pelvis is trimmed if needed. The UPJ and the trimmed part of the pelvis remain undismembered and are removed only after the last suture is placed, thus maintaining stability and decreasing tension on the suture line. The stent is left indwelling for 4 to 6 weeks. The Foley catheter is removed 24 hours after surgery. The children are covered with prophylactic antibiotics.

Results

It is well known that adhering to sound surgical principles, minimal handling of the ureter at the time of repair, and judicious use of internal stenting or nephrostomy tube drainage ensures a successful outcome.[2] A successful pyeloplasty has been defined as improvement in hydronephrosis and stabilization or improvement in function on renal scan along with a decrease in washout time. In those situations where the child presents with symptoms, resolution of flank/abdominal pain or vomiting should also occur.[2] Several series have reported good results following laparoscopic pyeloplasty (**Table 1**).

Laparoscopic pyeloplasty offers substantial benefits to children by decreasing morbidity, accelerating postoperative recovery, causing less pain, and improving cosmetic outcome. Multiple series have demonstrated high success rates (92%–100%) and low perioperative morbidity, although only a few consist of cohorts of more than 100 cases.

Laparoscopic pyeloplasty in comparison with open pyeloplasty

Open pyeloplasty has remained the gold standard in the management of UPJ obstruction in both adult and pediatric populations. The success rates

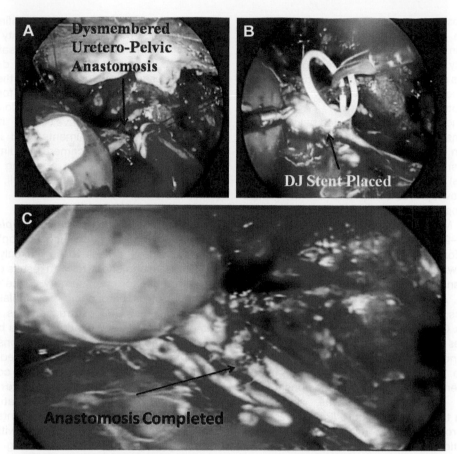

Fig. 5. Retroperitoneal laparoscopic pyeloplasty. (*A*) Posterior Ureteropelvic anastomosis being made. (*B*) Double-J (DJ) stent placed. (*C*) Anastomosis completed.

of open pyeloplasty have been reported to be 90% to 100%.[13,14] However, open surgical pyeloplasty results in significant perioperative and postoperative morbidity, postoperative pain, and scar formation.

Soulie and colleagues[15] compared retroperitoneal laparoscopic with open pyeloplasty with a minimal incision in 53 consecutive nonrandomized adults. The mean operating time (165 vs 145 minutes) was similar in both groups. Incidence of complications, hospital stay, and functional results were equivalent for both groups, but the return to painless activity was more rapid with laparoscopy in younger patients. Ravish and colleagues[16] reported their experience in 29 patients with a mean operative time of 159 minutes in open pyeloplasty and 214 minutes in laparoscopic pyeloplasty. Although pain scores were lower in

Table 1
Laparoscopic dismembered pyeloplasty in children

Authors,[Ref.] Year	No. of Cases	Age (y)	OT (min)	Conversion Rate (%)	Complication Rate (%)	SR (%)
Reddy et al,[8] 2005	16	3.5	160	0	6.25	100
Lopez et al,[9] 2009	32	7.7	152	9.3	10.3	100
Metzelder et al,[10] 2006	46	5.5	175	4.3	6.8	96
Vincentini et al,[11] 2008	23	3.75	175–180	0	0	100
Sweeney et al,[12] 2011	112	9.4	254	0.8	10.8	97

Abbreviations: OT, operative time; SR, success rate.
Data from Refs.[8–12]

the laparoscopic group on postoperative days 1 and 2, no child from either group required pain medication after 72 hours. The difference was not statistically significant between the 2 groups. One failure was noted in the laparoscopic group, which was successfully managed by retrograde endopyelotomy.

Penn and colleagues[17] evaluated outcomes between transperitoneal laparoscopic and open pyeloplasty in children. Twenty children (mean age 7.8 years) underwent laparoscopy while 19 (7.2 years) underwent open surgery ($P = .48$). Mean follow-up was similar between the groups (laparoscopic 8.1 months vs open 11.1 months, $P = .38$). Mean operative time was 151 minutes (range 94–213) for laparoscopy and 130 minutes (83–225) for open surgery ($P = .09$). Mean hospitalization was 29.3 hours (range 20.5–48) for laparoscopy and 36.2 hours (24–73) for open surgery ($P = .06$). Analgesic usage was similar between the groups. One failure in the open arm required a revision. Operative, hospital, anesthetic, and total charges were similar between the groups.

Tong and colleagues[18] reported on 23 infants aged 2 to 12 months (mean 7.3 months) undergoing open pyeloplasty or retroperitoneal laparoscopy. Operative time was significantly shorter in the open procedure (95 minutes) than with laparoscopy (102.6 minutes). Success and complication rates were similar between the 2 groups, but hospitalization and return of bowel function were significantly shorter in the laparoscopic group. Incision length was also statistically shorter following laparoscopic pyeloplasty (2 cm) versus open pyeloplasty (5 cm). This study particularly looked at this age group (infants) because some consider that there would be no advantage in incision size, and a more conspicuous incision is noted with the dorsal lumbotomy approach.

Bonnard and colleagues[19] were probably the first to report on retroperitoneal laparoscopic versus open pyeloplasty in children. A total of 22 children with a mean age of 88 months (range 25–192 months) underwent laparoscopic dismembered pyeloplasty via a retroperitoneal approach. An additional 17 children with a mean age of 103 months (range 37–206 months) underwent similar procedures via open surgery through a flank incision. The 2 groups were similar in mean age and weight. The mean operative time was significantly shorter in the open surgery than in the laparoscopy group: 96 minutes (range 50–150 minutes) versus 219 minutes (range 140–310 minutes). Mean use of acetaminophen and morphine derivatives was less in the laparoscopy group, and the mean hospital stay was shorter. All these studies confirmed the feasibility of laparoscopic pyeloplasty even in younger children, in addition to safety and decreased morbidity in the form of decreased analgesic use and hospital stay. As these were earlier studies, the operating time for laparoscopic pyeloplasty was significantly longer than for open surgery. However, with increased experience, better instruments, and improved vision (high-definition camera, 3-dimensional camera and monitors), the operating times of laparoscopy have decreased (RB Nerli, 2014 unpublished data).

Complications of laparoscopic pyeloplasty

Over the past 2 decades laparoscopic pyeloplasty has proved itself to be not only feasible but also safe and effective, with results comparable with those for open surgery. Since the introduction of laparoscopic pyeloplasty, the management of UPJ obstruction has gradually witnessed substantial changes and is becoming more commonly applied. Complications of laparoscopic pyeloplasty series published to date include prolonged drainage and ileus, conversion to an open procedure, postoperative nephrectomy, urinary tract infection, hematuria, and displaced double-pigtail ureteral stents.[2,20] Potential intraoperative complications with laparoscopic pyeloplasty include bleeding requiring transfusion, trocar damage to viscera or vessels, and thermal damage to tissues or organs.[2,20] A rare, but significant, complication is bowel injury, the risk of which might be higher if a transperitoneal or even a transmesenteric access is used. Occasionally, a double-pigtail ureteral stent cannot be advanced into the bladder and urethroscopic repositioning of the stent might become necessary. Potential postoperative complications include hernia internally or at the port site, wound infection, persistent urine leakage, and urinary tract infection. Postoperative ileus is a complication with the transperitoneal approach, owing to leakage of urine from the anastomosis.[2]

Based on their experience with 103 cases of laparoscopic pyeloplasty in children, Nerli and colleagues[20] reported on the complications and the definitive learning curve. Intraoperative incidents occurred in 2.91% of the cases, mostly without consequences for the child, including faulty port placement, needing placement of an extra port, and umbilical port side bleed. Postoperative complications occurred in 11.65% of children and included prolonged ileus, prolonged urinary leak, fever, hematuria, and recurrent UPJ stenosis, which occurred in 4.85% of children needing reoperation.

ROBOT-ASSISTED LAPAROSCOPIC PYELOPLASTY

The introduction of laparoscopy allowed for minimally invasive reconstructive surgery that mirrored open surgical procedures. These techniques offer substantial benefits to patients by decreasing morbidity, accelerating postoperative recovery, causing less pain, and improving cosmetic outcome. However, several experts believe that laparoscopic pyeloplasty is a difficult operation to master, more so in children. The major difficulty of laparoscopic pyeloplasty is intracorporeal suturing, which prolongs operative times,[21,22] and the relatively steep learning curve for this procedure because of the technical difficulties of suturing and anastomosis. On the other hand, robotics has several advantages in complex laparoscopic reconstructive procedures such as pyeloplasty. Using the da Vinci robotic system, all steps of traditional Anderson-Hynes dismembered pyeloplasty can be performed.[21,23] The advantages of the da Vinci robot include tremor control, 1:5 motion scaling, 6° of freedom within 1 cm of the tip of the end effector, true 3-dimensional vision, simplified suturing, and improved operative technique.

The da Vinci Surgical System (Intuitive Surgical, Mountain View, CA, USA) was approved by the Food and Drug Administration to perform laparoscopic procedures in July 2000. It is a master-slave robot that integrates a comfortable surgeon console with a portable patient side cart consisting of a camera arm and 2 robotic instrument arms. The unique instrument "wrists" have 7° of freedom, which eliminate the long fulcrum of standard laparoscopic instruments that tends to exaggerate movements in pelvic laparoscopy. The robotic arms move in the same direction as the surgeon's hands, in contrast to conventional laparoscopic instruments. Subsequent modification of the patient side cart now also offers an optional third instrument arm or "fourth arm," which can be used to aid in retraction.[24] The da Vinci optics include 6× to 10× magnification and 3-dimensional stereoscopic visualization, which allows for improved depth and shadow perception. The improved depth perception allows for more rapid and precise fine movements such as suture placement. Other advantages that improve precision include tremor filtering and motion scaling. Finally, the comfortable sitting position at the surgeon console helps to reduce surgeon fatigue, a significant factor in laparoscopic cases with long operative times that require focus and concentration for accurate intracorporeal suturing.

Gettman and colleagues[25] were the first to report a series of 9 patients who underwent Anderson-Hynes robotic-assisted laparoscopic pyeloplasty in 2002. At 4 months' follow-up, the success rate was 89%. However, 1 patient required open repair of a renal pelvis leak. Yohannes and Burjonrappa[26] also reported a single case of successful robotic-assisted laparoscopic pyeloplasty shortly after Gettman's initial report. Although operative time was prolonged (5 hours), they completed the procedure successfully with no complications. Gettman and colleagues[27] compared 6 robotic-assisted laparoscopic pyeloplasties with 6 standard laparoscopic pyeloplasties, using either an Anderson-Hynes or a Fenger technique in each group. Use of the robot was found to significantly decrease both operative and anastomotic time, especially in the Anderson-Hynes group.

Robotic-assisted surgery (RAS) was gradually introduced into managing pediatric urologic problems, and has the possibility to overcome many impediments of conventional laparoscopic surgery and decrease the learning curve for MIS, especially for pediatric reconstructive procedures.[28] RAS also allows the seasoned laparoscopist to become more proficient and refined, providing a larger "tool box" with which to expand MIS to more complex reconstructive procedures. The procedure most performed in pediatric urology is pyeloplasty for UPJ obstruction.

Comparison of Laparoscopic Pyeloplasty with Robot-Assisted Laparoscopic Pyeloplasty

The use of robotic assistance in urologic laparoscopy has expanded exponentially in recent years, given the unique features provided by the robotic platform, especially in the setting of reconstructive procedures where extensive suturing is needed. Autorino and colleagues[29] critically analyzed the current status of laparoscopic and robotic repair of UPJ obstruction by systematically reviewing literature using PubMed. Article selection proceeded according to the search strategy based on Preferred Reporting Items for Systematic Reviews and Meta-analyses criteria. Multiple series of laparoscopic pyeloplasty demonstrated high success rates and low perioperative morbidity in pediatric populations with both the transperitoneal and retroperitoneal approaches (**Table 2**). Data on pediatric robot-assisted pyeloplasty were increasingly becoming available. Robot-assisted redo pyeloplasty was mostly described in the pediatric population. Internal-external stenting as well as a stentless approach had been used, especially in the pediatric population. Comparative studies demonstrated similar success and complication rates between minimally invasive and open

Table 2
Robot-assisted laparoscopic pyeloplasty in children

Authors,[Ref.] Year	Approach	No. of Cases	Age (y)	OT (min)	Complication Rate (%)	SR (%)
Olsen et al,[30] 2007	Retro	67	7.9	146	17.9	94
Minnillo et al,[31] 2011	Trans	155	10.5	198.5	11	96
Singh et al,[32] 2012	Trans	34	12	105	8.8	97

Abbreviations: OT, operative time; Retro, retroperitoneal; SR, success rate; Trans, transperitoneal.
   Data from Refs.[30–32]

pyeloplasty in the pediatric setting. The investigators concluded that laparoscopy represented an efficient and effective minimally invasive alternative to open pyeloplasty. Robotic pyeloplasty was likely to emerge as the new minimally invasive standard of care whenever robotic technology was available, because its precise suturing and shorter learning curve represented unique attractive features. For both laparoscopy and robotics, the technique could be tailored to the specific case according to intraoperative findings and personal surgical experience.

Role of Laparoscopic Pyeloplasty in the Robotic Era

It is now well known that robotic-assisted surgery offers several advantages over traditional laparoscopy, including 3-dimensional visualization and 7° of wrist movement. These specific robotic properties allow for easier dissection of the renal pelvis in addition to precise trimming and reconstruction of the UPJ.[24] In 2003, Gettman and colleagues[27] reported shorter overall operative and anastomotic times with da Vinci robotic pyeloplasty in adults. The main disadvantage of the da Vinci Surgical System is its high cost.

With ever increasing advantages of the RAS, the disadvantages of traditional laparoscopic procedures become highlighted. The disadvantages associated with laparoscopic procedures are mainly due to the nonergonomic design of surgical instruments and outdated environment of operating theaters. Today laparoscopic surgery has become more advanced, operating time has expanded, and, in proportion, so have the levels of mental and physical stress imposed on the surgical team.[33,34] However, only minor changes have been made to the theater originally designed for conventional operations. Apart from poor ergonomics, laparoscopy is also handicapped by reduction of the range of motion caused by the fixed trocar position determining the angle of the respective instrument to the working field. The

incision point acts like a spherical joint that limits the degrees of freedom of the instrument from 6 to only 4: jaw, pitch, rotation, and insertion, plus the actuation of instrument.[35] Other problems of laparoscopy include the 2-dimensional view of the telescope, absence of shadows, stereovision, and movement parallax, which in particular makes it difficult to accurately determine spatial distance and movements, thus impairing eye-hand coordination.[36]

These drawbacks bring up the question, "What is the role of laparoscopic pyeloplasty in the robotic era?" Laparoscopic pyeloplasty is here to stay because of its advantages of safety, efficacy, decreased morbidity, reduced hospital stay, and cost-effectiveness compared with robotic-assisted laparoscopic pyeloplasty. Autorino and colleagues[29] systematically reviewed several series of laparoscopic and robotic repair of UPJ obstruction, and reported that laparoscopic pyeloplasty demonstrated high success rates and low perioperative morbidity in pediatric populations. Comparative studies of laparoscopic and robot-assisted repairs demonstrated similar success rates.

One of the major disadvantages of robot-assisted surgery is the cost of the procedure. In India, for example, the costs associated with laparoscopic pyeloplasty would be nearly 20% of the cost of robotic-assisted laparoscopic pyeloplasty. The cost differential could be significant in many other countries where, similar to India, most health care costs are borne by the patient rather than through a third-party payor system.[37,38] Laparoscopic surgery would benefit from significant improvements in ergonomics, such as a chair for the surgeon, specially designed operating room tables, and ergonomically designed instrument handles. Future modifications of the laparoscopic technique, such as a single-port surgery (eg, laparoendoscopic single-site surgery), may also have an impact on the application and use of laparoscopic pyeloplasty.[39]

STEPS TO OVERCOME LIMITATIONS OF LAPAROSCOPIC PYELOPLASTY

Several steps[40] need to be taken to address the ergonomic limitations of laparoscopy so as to reduce the disadvantages associated with laparoscopic procedures:

- Adjustable operating table to guarantee relaxed working (ie, right angle of elbow)
- Seating arrangement to enable the surgeon to operate temporarily in a seated position
- Specialized chairs that incorporate pedal switches and body support (eg, cockpit type) to reduce fatigue
- Adjustable monitor height to avoid "chin-up" position
- Semilunar arrangement of trocars to provide an adequate angle
- Use of a motorized camera holder (voice/motion controlled) to improve the stability of the image
- Insertion of instruments by the operating room nurse/assistants, enabling the surgeon to keep his or her eye on the monitor
- Participation in a trunk endurance training program (the surgeon needs to exercise arm and back muscles with yoga and relaxation techniques)

Several visual aids have been described to improve the surgeon's depth perception. Shadows can be introduced by using illumination cannulae. Stereovision can be introduced by using a stereoendoscopic system.[40] Another possibility would be the use of flexible endoscopes and instruments. By contrast, the recent introduction of high-definition television technology has significantly improved depth perception, mainly resulting from better resolution of the image.[39]

SUMMARY

Laparoscopic pyeloplasty is here to stay because of its advantages of safety, efficacy, decreased morbidity, reduced hospital stay, and significant cost-effectiveness in comparison with robotic-assisted laparoscopic pyeloplasty. Laparoscopic surgery would benefit from significant improvements in ergonomics, such as a chair for the surgeon, specially designed operating room tables, and ergonomically designed instrument handles. Future modifications of the laparoscopic technique, such as single-port surgery (eg, laparoendoscopic single-site surgery), may also have an impact on the application and use of laparoscopic pyeloplasty.

REFERENCES

1. Brown T, Mandell J, Lebowitz RL. Neonatal hydronephrosis in the era of sonography. AJR Am J Roentgenol 1987;148:959–63.
2. Carr MC, Casale P. Anomalies and surgery of the ureter in children. In: Wein AJ, Kavoussi LR, Novick AC, et al, editors. Campbell-Walsh urology. 10th edition. Philadelphia: Elsevier Saunders; 2012. p. 3212–35.
3. Kavoussi LR, Peters CA. Laparoscopic pyeloplasty. J Urol 1993;150:1891.
4. Schuessler WW, Grune MT, Tecuanhuey LV, et al. Laparoscopic dismembered pyeloplasty. J Urol 1993;150:1795.
5. Tan H. Laparoscopic Anderson-Hynes dismembered pyeloplasty in children. J Urol 1999;162:1045.
6. Yeung CK, Tam YH, Sihoe JD, et al. Retroperitoneoscopic dismembered pyeloplasty for pelviureteric junction obstruction in infants and children. Br J Urol 2001;87:509.
7. El Ghoneimi A, Farhat W, Bolduc S, et al. Laparoscopic dismembered pyeloplasty by a retroperitoneal approach in children. BJU Int 2003;92:104.
8. Reddy M, Nerli RB, Bashetty R, et al. Laparoscopic dismembered pyeloplasty in children. J Urol 2005;174:700–2.
9. Lopez M, Guye E, Becmeur F, et al. Laparoscopic pyeloplasty for repair of pelviureteric junction obstruction in children. J Laparoendosc Adv Surg Tech A 2009;19(Suppl 1):S91–3.
10. Metzelder ML, Schier F, Petersen C, et al. Laparoscopic transabdominal pyeloplasty in children is feasible irrespective of age. J Urol 2006;175:688–91.
11. Vicentini FC, Dé nes FT, Borges LL, et al. Laparoscopic pyeloplasty in children: is the outcome different in children under 2 years of age? J Pediatr Urol 2008;4:348–51.
12. Sweeney DD, Ost MC, Schneck FX, et al. Laparoscopic pyeloplasty for ureteropelvic junction obstruction in children. J Laparoendosc Adv Surg Tech A 2011;21:261–5.
13. Notley RG, Beaurgie JM. The long term follow up of Anderson-Hynes pyeloplasty for hydronephrosis. Br J Urol 1973;45:464.
14. Perksy L, Kraurse JR, Boltuch RL. Initial complications and late results in dismembered pyeloplasty. J Urol 1977;118:162.
15. Soulie M, Thoulouzan M, Seguin P, et al. Retroperitoneal laparoscopic versus open pyeloplasty with a minimal incision; Comparison of two surgical approaches. Urology 2001;57:443.
16. Ravish IR, Nerli RB, Reddy MN, et al. Laparoscopic pyeloplasty compared with open pyeloplasty in children. J Endourol 2007;21:897–901.
17. Penn HA, Gatti JM, Hoestje SM, et al. Laparoscopic versus open pyeloplasty in children: preliminary

report of a prospective randomized trial. J Urol 2010;184:690–5.

18. Tong Q, Zheng L, Tang S, et al. Comparison of laparoscopic-assisted versus open dismembered pyeloplasty for ureteropelvic junction obstruction in infants: intermediate results. Urology 2009;74:889.

19. Bonnard A, Fouquet V, Carricaburu E, et al. Retroperitoneoscopic laparoscopic versus open pyeloplasty in children. J Urol 2005;173:1710.

20. Nerli RB, Reddy M, Prabha V, et al. Complications of laparoscopic pyeloplasty in children. Pediatr Surg Int 2009;25:343–7.

21. Janetschek G, Peschel R, Frauscher F. Laparoscopic pyeloplasty. Urol Clin North Am 2000;27:695.

22. Chen RN, Moore RG, Kavoussi LR. Laparoscopic pyeloplasty. Indications, technique, and long-term outcome. Urol Clin North Am 1998;25:323.

23. Olsen LH, Jorgensen TM. Computer assisted pyeloplasty in children: the retroperitoneal approach. J Urol 2004;171:2629.

24. Atug F, Woods M, Burgess SV, Castle EP, Thomas R. Robotic assisted laparoscopic pyeloplasty in children. J Urol 2005;174:1440–2.

25. Gettman M, Neururer R, Bartsch G, et al. Anderson-Hynes dismembered pyeloplasty performed using the da Vinci robotic system. Urology 2002; 60:509–13.

26. Yohannes P, Burjonrappa S. Laparoscopic Anderson-Hynes dismembered pyeloplasty using the da Vinci robot: technical considerations. J Endourol 2003;17: 79–83.

27. Gettman M, Peschel R, Neururer R, et al. A comparison of laparoscopic pyeloplasty performed with the da Vinci robotic system versus standard laparoscopic techniques: initial clinical results. Eur Urol 2002;42: 453–8.

28. Casale P, Kojima Y. Robotic-assisted laparoscopic surgery in pediatric urology: an update. Scand J Surg 2009;98:110–9.

29. Autorino R, Eden C, El Ghoneimi A, et al. Robot-assisted and laparoscopic repair of ureteropelvic junction obstruction: a systematic review and meta-analysis. Eur Urol 2014;65:430–52.

30. Olsen LH, Rawashdeh YF, Jorgensen TM. Pediatric robot assisted retroperitoneoscopic pyeloplasty: a 5-year experience. J Urol 2007;178: 2137–41.

31. Minnillo BJ, Cruz JA, Sayao RH, et al. Long-term experience and outcomes of robotic assisted laparoscopic pyeloplasty in children and young adults. J Urol 2011;185:1455–60.

32. Singh P, Dogra PN, Kumar R, et al. Outcomes of robot-assisted laparoscopic pyeloplasty in children: a single center experience. J Endourol 2012;26: 249–53.

33. Vereczkel A, Bupp H, Feussner H. Laparoscopic surgery and ergonomics—it's time to think on ourselves as well. Surg Endosc 2003; 17:1680–2.

34. Hemal AK, Srinivas M, Charles AR. Ergonomic problems associated with laparoscopy. J Endourol 2001; 15:499–503.

35. Rassweiler J, Binder J, Frede T. Robotic and telesurgery: will they change our future? Curr Opin Urol 2001;11:309–20.

36. Breedveld P, Stassen HG, Meijer DW, et al. Theoretical background and conceptual solution for depth perception and eye-hand coordination problems in laparoscopic surgery. Minim Invasive Ther Allied Technol 1999;8:227–34.

37. Link RE, Bhayani SB, Kavoussi LR. A prospective comparison of robotic and laparoscopic pyeloplasty. Ann Surg 2006;243(4):486.

38. Braga LH, Pace K, DeMaria J, et al. Systematic review and meta-analysis of robotic-assisted versus conventional laparoscopic pyeloplasty for patients with ureteropelvic junction obstruction: effect on operative time, length of hospital stay, postoperative complications, and success rate. Eur Urol 2009; 56(5):848–58.

39. Rassweiler J, Hruza M, Klein J, et al. The role of laparoscopic radical prostatectomy in the era of robotic surgery. Eur Urol Suppl 2010;9(3):379–87.

40. Schurr MO, Kunert W, Arezzo A, et al. The role and future of endoscopic imaging systems. Endoscopy 1999;71:557–62.

Vesicoscopic Ureteral Reimplant
Is There a Role in the Age of Robotics?

Megan S. Schober, MD, PhD, Venkata R. Jayanthi, MD*

KEYWORDS

- Vesicoscopic reimplant • Vesicoureteral reflux • Ureteral reimpantation

KEY POINTS

- Vesicoscopic reimplant is a minimally invasive procedure for the definitive repair of primary reflux.
- Although technically challenging to learn, vesicoscopic reimplant success rates are equivalent to open and robotic-assisted repair after the learning curve is endured.
- Vesicoscopic reimplant is a technique that is used in patients with the standard indications for surgical treatment of vesicoureteral reflux.
- Patients that may require extensive ureteral tapering or have a very small bladder capacity are not good candidates for vesicoscopic reimplant.
- There is an economic benefit to vesicoscopic reimplant when compared with robotic assisted laparoscopic ureteral reimplant.

 A video of vesicoscopic ureteral reimpantation accompanies this article at http://www.urologic. theclinics.com/

INTRODUCTION

Vesicoscopic ureteral reimplantation (VUR) is a relatively common clinical problem in children that is characterized by the retrograde flow of urine from the bladder to the upper urinary tracts. The true prevalence of reflux is difficult to accurately assess because it can be completely asymptomatic. In children with prenatal hydronephrosis, the presence of VUR ranges from 15% in children with little or no residual postnatal hydronephrosis to 38% in children who are found to have significant hydronephrosis or other upper tract anomalies.[1,2] Multiple studies have shown that between 68% and 85% of grade I to II VUR will spontaneously resolve and grade III VUR will resolve in about 50% of patients.[3–6]

Approaches to intervention are varied and range from endoscopic injection at the ureterovesical junction to open surgical correction. Dextranomer/hyaluronic acid is a common endoscopic treatment of VUR in the United States. Published success rates of this method range from 68% (duplex ureters) to 89% depending on grade of reflux.[7–9] Historically, open ureteral reimplant has been the gold standard in treatment of VUR with a success rate approaching 100%.[10,11] There are multiple minimally invasive surgical options for correction of reflux including purely laparoscopic, robotic-assisted, or endoscopic approaches.

Pure laparoscopic ureteral reimplant using the extravesical approach (LEVUR) has been performed with good results. LEVUR was first

---

Section of Pediatric Urology, Nationwide Children's Hospital, 700 Children's Dr., Columbus, OH 43215, USA
* Corresponding author.
E-mail address: Rama.Jayanthi@nationwidechildrens.org

Urol Clin N Am 42 (2015) 53–59
http://dx.doi.org/10.1016/j.ucl.2014.09.005

performed in a porcine model in 1993, and shortly thereafter, Ehrlich and colleagues[12] performed this surgery in children.[13] In a series of 81 patients in a multi-institutional study, Riquelme and colleagues[14] demonstrated a 95.8% rate of VUR resolution on follow-up imaging after LEVUR. Robotic-assisted extravesical ureteral reimplant (RALUR) has been steadily gaining popularity in pediatric urology. Multiple series have been published demonstrating outcomes of RALUR similar to those of open surgery.[15] However, these studies have also shown a significant disparity in the cost and operative times between robotic and open ureteral reimplantation.[16,17] One series also demonstrated that the rate of complications was similar between robotic and open reimplant, but the Clavien grade of complication was higher in the robotic group and included ureteral stenosis and urine leak.[18]

Intravesical RALUR is not routinely performed at this time. The working space within the bladder is quite small, making robotic assistance more challenging in this scenario. Published series of intravesical RALUR are few, and patient follow-up is short.[19,20] As robotic systems currently available continue to evolve, intravesical RALUR may gain popularity in the future. A traditional advantage to intravesical versus extravesical approaches to ureteral reimplant is the decreased risk of postoperative bladder dysfunction, in particular, urinary retention. Nerve-sparing modifications to extravesical ureteral reimplant have been described in both the open and the robotic surgical literature. These modifications to surgical technique and dissection decrease the incidence of postoperative urinary retention.[21,22]

The idea of minimally invasive intravesical surgery to treat VUR is not new. In 1995, Okamura and colleagues[23] described a technique that used both cystoscopic and laparoscopic instrumentation to perform a trigonoplasty. In this procedure, the trigone is resected in a "fanwise" fashion and the ureteral orifices were brought medially by reapproximating the lateral aspects of the trigone with extracorporeal suturing. Follow-up studies of this procedure, however, demonstrated poor rates of reflux resolution in children when compared with adults undergoing the same procedure. Postoperatively, the pediatric patients in these series tended to have trigonal splitting resulting in the return of reflux in 41% of patients. Other drawbacks to this technique included long operative times, including a case that took 6 hours secondary to continued loss of insufflation and difficult visualization.

In 2001, Gill and colleagues[24] described a minimally invasive intravesical technique for VUR correction. The technique was first detailed in a published series of 3 patients. The procedure used glycine irrigation within the bladder and an electrosurgical Collins knife to perform a transurethral detrusor incision. After the detrusor incision is made, a submucosal cross-trigonal trough is made with laparoscopic instruments. The ureters are mobilized intravesically and brought across the trigone and secured in the submucosal tunnels by closing the bladder mucosal flaps over the ureters. Continuous bladder irrigation was used to provide bladder distention and visualization during the surgery. This method introduced intracorporeal suturing to intravesical ureteral reimplantation as well as ureteral dissection.

Yeung and colleagues[25] modified the procedure in 2005 and, instead of glycine irrigation, the bladder was insufflated with carbon dioxide mimicking traditional laparoscopy. The initial published report of this technique included 16 patients with a 96% rate of reflux resolution. Multiple groups have demonstrated good results with this technique. In 2006, a series of 32 patients undergoing vesicoscopic reimplantation (VR) was reported by Kutikov and colleagues.[26] In this series, 92.6% of patients had resolution of VUR; however, there was a relatively high complication rate with postoperative urine leak in 12.5% and ureteral stricture in 6.3% of patients. Importantly, this study showed that most of complications were encountered in patients less than 2 years of age or with a bladder capacity less than 130 mL. This study established the importance of patient selection with the VR technique. In 2007, the authors published a series of 52 children who underwent VR.[27] In their initial series, reflux resolution was 91% in the VR patients compared with 97% in patients who underwent open ureteral reimplantation. The analgesic requirements were less in the VR group, and patients also subjectively described less discomfort. In the authors' updated 2008 series of 100 patients, 94% of patients who underwent postoperative imaging had complete resolution of reflux.[28] Improvement in the success rate of the surgery is attributed to increased surgeon experience with VR as well as technical adjustments to the procedure over time. Valla and colleagues[29] also published encouraging results with the VR technique in 2009, demonstrating a success rate of 92% in 72 patients with primary VUR. VR has been established as a good option for surgical repair of VUR requiring correction. The authors' extended experience of 167 patients who have undergone VR is presented here.

INDICATIONS/CONTRAINDICATIONS

VR at the authors' institution is performed on children older than 4 years. The authors have found that older children benefit the most from this procedure and the intravesical space is typically sufficient in this age group. Because VR is technically demanding and involves complex reconstruction in a limited space, the authors continue to be selective in offering VR to patients in whom no ureteral tapering is anticipated. Most children who underwent the procedure were between 5 and 6 years of age with persistent VUR or symptomatic urinary tract infection. In children with grade IV VUR, VR was offered only if ureteral tapering was thought to be unlikely. Ureteral duplication is not considered a contraindication to VR. Patients with duplex ureters underwent common sheath VR.

TECHNIQUE
Anesthesia

A standard anesthetic protocol was performed with a combination of inhaled and intravenous anesthetic agents (Video 1). Caudal epidural anesthesia was administered after anesthesia induction for patients who had consented. Ketorolac was given before the end of the procedure and then given every 6 hours postoperatively while patients were admitted to the hospital. For breakthrough pain, opioids were given and oxybutynin was administered to children as needed for abdominal pain suggestive of bladder spasm.

Cystoscopy and Bladder Wall Fixation

A 30° lens rigid cystocope is inserted into the urethra and the bladder is drained. Once the bladder is empty, CO_2 insufflation is initiated via the cystoscope while the vesicoscopic ports are placed. After adequate bladder distention is achieved, the ports are placed under direct cystoscopic vision. The first step in port placement is to anchor the anterior bladder wall to the abdominal wall. This method is modified from a technique first described to repair inguinal hernias laparoscopically in children[30]; this is achieved by loading a 2-0 polydioxanone suture with the needle cut off through an 18-gauge spinal needle. The needle is passed into the bladder through the anterior abdominal wall under direct vision. The suture is advanced into the bladder, forming a loop. The spinal needle is removed and replaced into the bladder guiding it through the loop of suture. The tail of the suture is then passed through the spinal needle and the suture is advanced through the loop. The 2 ends of the suture outside the

abdomen are then pulled up, thus pulling the end of the suture outside the body. The suture is then tied to anchor the bladder to the abdominal wall. Three fixation sutures are placed immediately proximal to the points where ports will be placed. Ideally, the ports should be placed as cranially as possible without traversing the peritoneum. There is potential for bowel injury if the port enters the peritoneum; however, if the peritoneum is traversed without bowel injury, the procedure can proceed but the resultant pneumoperitoneum may inhibit visibility and distort the bladder. If visibility and bladder anatomy are affected by pneumoperitoneum, a Veress needle can be placed in the umbilicus to help decompress the abdomen. The added step of bladder fixation to the anterior abdominal wall before port placement helps to provide adequate resistance to allow the ports to be easily introduced into the otherwise freely mobile bladder.

Port Placement

Ports are placed in a triangulated fashion in the lower abdomen. A 5-mm port is placed in the midline for the 5-mm 30° lens camera. Two 3-mm ports are placed laterally and at a slightly caudal position to the camera port. The ports are placed adjacent to the points previously fixed to the anterior abdominal wall. This arrangement provides a comfortable working angle at the depth of the bladder base. For most children, 3 mm × 20 cm laparoscopic instruments are ideal.

Ureteral Dissection

A 3.5-Fr feeding tube is precut to an appropriate size for the patient. A good rule of thumb is to add 10 to the patient's age and cut the tube to that number of centimeters. A 5-0 polydioxanone suture is used to fix the feeding tube to the ureteral orifice. In female patients, one can preload the suture onto the feeding tube 2 cm proximal to the end of the tube before inserting it into the urethra, thereby eliminating a step in the intracorporeal suturing process. Once the tube is in place, the hook cautery electrode on low power is used to demarcate a cuff of mucosa around the ureteral orifice. The ureter is then dissected into the bladder along this space, analogous to an open intravesical ureteral reimplant. Gentle traction is maintained on the fixation suture, allowing the planes to be easily visualized. Both sharp and blunt dissection are used and care must be taken when transecting bands of investing detrusor muscle off of the ureter. It is sometimes best to divide these bands sharply. In children with thin-walled bladders, this dissection can be achieved quickly; however, in children with thick-walled bladders, the dissection can be difficult and cumbersome. The dissection is complete when the freed ureter can reach the contralateral side of the bladder. The posterior detrusorotomy can then be closed with interrupted 4-0 polydioxanone suture using intracorporeal laparoscopic suturing technique. For bilateral re-implantation, the contralateral side can now be mobilized. To aid in visualization, a 3-mm irrigation suction device can be used to remove blood or urine through the working ports as needed. Some authors have advocated leaving a small urethral catheter in place during the procedure to help in this regard, but the authors have found this unnecessary.

Tunnel Creation

The tunnel is then created beginning from the initial hiatus toward the contralateral side. Maryland grasping forceps are used to elevate the mucosa, and fine scissors are used to initiate the plane. The tunnel is created with both sharp and blunt dissection. Once the tunnel has been created, the feeding tube within the ureter is used to help guide the ureter through the tunnel. The ureteral orifice is then sutured in position at the new hiatus with interrupted 5-0 polydioxanone suture. The remaining mucosal openings are closed, and the feeding tubes are removed.

Port Closure

A 5-Fr feeding tube is passed through each port site as it is closed to maintain the pathway through the incision into the bladder. In a manner similar to the bladder fixation step, the bladder mucosa is closed with 2-0 polydioxanone suture through an 18-gauge spinal needle. However, when the bladder mucosa is closed, care is taken not to go incorporate the fascia, allowing the bladder to fall away from the abdominal wall. The bladder wall sutures are then carefully tied and the skin incisions are closed with 5-0 polyglactin suture. A Foley catheter is placed at the end of the procedure and left to dependent drainage.

Postoperative Care

Patients are admitted to the surgical floor post-procedure and are continued on appropriate perioperative intravenous antibiotics for 3 post-operative doses or until discharge, which is typically the following morning. Antibiotic choice may differ in light of patient allergies or profile of prior positive urine cultures. Patients are started on a clear liquid diet immediately after surgery and diet is advanced as tolerated. The Foley catheter is generally removed the morning after

surgery. Reasons to keep the Foley catheter in place longer than this include significant gross hematuria, excessively difficult ureteral dissection, or abnormally thickened bladder wall. Ketorolac and acetaminophen are used for pain control and hydrocodone/acetaminophen is used for any breakthrough pain. Oxybutynin is also used to limit bladder spasm. Patients will also be kept on polyethylene glycol in the immediate postoperative period as well because a great number of these patients also have significant constipation issues.

Follow-up

Antibiotic prophylaxis is continued for the first month after reimplantation. A follow-up office visit with a renal ultrasound is scheduled for 4 weeks after surgery. If renal ultrasound does not demonstrate any significant hydroureteronephrosis, prophylaxis is discontinued. Currently, voiding cystourethrogram (VCUG) is not performed if the patient is clinically doing well and there are no significant findings on renal ultrasound. No residual VUR was demonstrated on postoperative VCUG in 95% of the first 96 patients in the series. VCUG was offered to parents as an option after the first 96 patients in the series, but all parents declined.

COMPLICATIONS AND MANAGEMENT

Intraoperative complications encountered were associated with port placement. Pneumoperitoneum occurred occasionally and was treated by Veress needle placement during the procedure to "vent" the abdomen. By evacuating the abdomen in this fashion, the operation could proceed. During one early procedure, an inferior epigastric vessel was lacerated on port entry, causing a significant abdominal wall hematoma requiring open conversion of the procedure. There were 3 other open conversions early in the series all due to poor port placement. Ports in these cases were placed too caudally and therefore directly over the orifices, thus making dissection too difficult to complete vesicoscopically.

One patient developed a small extraperitoneal bladder leak postoperatively, which healed with catheter drainage. This complication occurred in a patient who did not have a formal closure of her bladder port sites. After this case, all port sites are formally closed and this complication has not been encountered again.

Two patients developed postoperative ureteral obstruction. Both patients initially underwent nephrostomy tube drainage. Imaging studies suggested extrinsic compression from retrovesical urinomas. One patient was successfully treated with temporary ureteral stenting and the second underwent reoperative ureteral reimplant at another center.

OUTCOMES

At the authors' institution, 167 children (151 girls, 16 boys) have undergone vesicoscopic ureteral reimplant by a single surgeon. Of these patients, 126 children underwent bilateral reimplantation. Mean operative time for a unilateral reimplant was 170.5 minutes and 194.0 minutes for bilateral reimplant. Initially, patients underwent a VCUG postoperatively. There was complete resolution of reflux in 91 of 96 patients who had a postoperative VCUG. Using resolution of reflux as an endpoint, this demonstrates a 95% success rate. Four of these patients were considered "true failures." These failures were all within the first 30 cases being performed and considered to be within the learning curve of the operation. Cystoscopy was performed in 3 of these patients and revealed ureterovesical fistulas in 2 and no intramural tunnel in one. One patient subsequently underwent injection therapy and the other 2 did not require any further treatment. One patient developed contralateral reflux. Bladder stones developed in 1 patient, which passed spontaneously. Of interest, another patient has had 2 episodes of obstructing ureteral calculi. During both of these episodes, the patient was able to pass the stones with only medical expulsion therapy with no surgical intervention.

CURRENT CONTROVERSIES/FUTURE CONSIDERATIONS

VR has not gained wide popularity as a treatment of VUR presumably because of the technically challenging nature of the procedure. The authors' series as well as others in the literature demonstrates that VR and open reimplant have similar success rates. The learning curve for this surgery is steep; however, a committed surgeon can learn and use this operation with good results. Over time, there was a noticeable decrease in operative times. RALUR is becoming more commonplace at pediatric urology programs. One advantage of robotics over pure laparoscopy is the ease with which one can suture intracorporeally. Most RALURs being performed at this time are extravesical. Very few centers have routinely performed intravesical RALUR. Peters and Woo[19] published a series in 2005 of 6 children between the ages of 5 and 15 years who underwent intravesical RALUR. In that series, 1 child had persistent reflux and

another child had a bladder leak. In 2011, Marchini and colleagues[20] compared the outcomes of intravesical and extravesical RALUR to open reimplant. In their series, they performed 19 intravesical RALUR and found a 21% rate of bladder leak and 5% rate of urinary retention. In the authors' current series of VR, postoperative bladder leak was identified in 1 patient (0.006%) and urinary retention was not encountered on catheter removal in the authors' patients. In patients who have undergone VR at the authors' institution, none have had de novo voiding dysfunction; this is a distinct advantage of VR over other surgical approaches to VUR.

Personal correspondence with surgeons who have performed intravesical RALUR confirms that it is technically more challenging than extravesical RALUR and is mostly due to the small working space of the bladder and the space needed for robotic instruments, especially 5-mm robotic instruments that require a larger intracorporeal space for proper articulation.[31] As robotic innovations continue to emerge, intravesical RALUR may become less technically challenging.

Economic analysis of the last 16 consecutive ureteral reimplants at the authors' institution (7 open, 5 vesicoscopic, and 9 robotic) revealed a statistically significant difference in the charges for vesicoscopic reimplant (mean $39,756) versus robotic-assisted reimplant (mean $58,641; $P = .0067$). The charge difference, however, between vesicoscopic and open ureteral reimplant (mean $37,629) was not significant ($P = .6587$). Charges include facility fees, operating room times, and anesthesia fees. Operative times may contribute to this cost disparity. This cost may also decrease after amortization of the robotic system. Although robotic-assisted surgery is becoming commonplace in the United States, on a global perspective it is unclear how much impact the robot will have secondary to its cost-prohibitive nature.

In Marchini's series of 19 intravesical RALUR, the mean operative time was 232.6 ± 37.4 minutes. The mean operative time in the authors' series for unilateral reimplant was 170.5 minutes and 194.0 minutes for bilateral reimplant. In the 2005 feasibility study of intravesical RALUR in 6 children by Peters and Woo, the operative times are not reported, only stating that the procedure took "slightly longer" than open reimplant. In the initial series by Yeung and colleagues, mean operative time for VR was 136 minutes. Overall, robotic assistance does appear to increase operative times and may be due to increased operating room setup time and robot positioning.

Many studies, mostly in the adult urology literature, have compared outcomes between robotic-assisted surgery and open surgery. Radical prostatectomy, cystectomy, and pyeloplasty are 3 surgical procedures that have been studied in detail in regard to benefits or disadvantages of robotic versus open approaches. Decreased hospitalization times and less need for blood transfusions are associated with robotic prostatectomy and cystectomy when compared with their open counterparts; however, there is still a significant disparity in cost of procedure and operative times.[32,33] Ureteral reimplant in general is a procedure that only in rare and unusual circumstances would require blood transfusion or extended hospitalization postoperatively. Therefore, the benefits of robotic assistance in this regard may not be of great significance when performing a pediatric ureteral reimplant. Recent trends have demonstrated an increasing number of robotic-assisted pyeloplasties being performed in the pediatric and adult populations. Although still performed less often than open or pure laparoscopic pyeloplasty, robotic-assisted pyeloplasty has been shown to have similar clinical outcomes and length of hospital stay.[34] A distinct advantage of robotic assistance in pyeloplasty surgery is the relative ease of intracorporeal suturing when compared with pure laparoscopy. Robotic suturing may also serve as a minor advantage in ureteral reimplantation; however, the degree of suturing required in reimplant surgery versus pyeloplasty is much less.

In terms of surgical technique, there is always a benefit in developing pure laparoscopic reconstructive skills because not all hospitals have robotic instrumentation. Another benefit to pure laparoscopy is in cases of robotic malfunction; one can maintain a minimally invasive strategy rather than converting to open.

SUMMARY

VR is a minimally invasive procedure for the definitive repair of primary vesicoureteral reflux. Although technically challenging to learn, success rates are equivalent to open and robotic-assisted ureteral reimplantation and the learning curve is traversed. It is a technique best used for children older than 4 years of age with the standard indications for surgical repair of VUR. Patients, however, that may require extensive ureteral tapering or have a very small bladder capacity are not good candidates for this procedure. There is an economic benefit to VR when compared with RALUR. Published operative times are generally similar or shorter in VR when compared with RALUR; however, open

ureteral reimplantation is generally accomplished in a much shorter time period than either RALUR or VR. The authors report a 95% rate of resolution of reflux in children with postoperative VCUG.

SUPPLEMENTARY DATA

Supplementary data related to this article can be found online at http://dx.doi.org/10.1016/j.ucl. 2014.09.005.

REFERENCES

1. Phan V, Traubici J, Hershenfield B, et al. Vesicoureteral reflux in infants with isolated antenatal hydronephrosis. Pediatr Nephrol 2003;18:1224–8.
2. Zerin JM, Ritchey ML, Chang AC. Incidental vesicoureteral reflux in neonates with antenatally detected hydronephrosis and other renal abnormalities. Radiology 1993;187(1):157–60.
3. Duckett JW. Vesicoureteral reflux: a 'conservative' analysis. Am J Kidney Dis 1983;3(2):139–44.
4. Arant BS Jr. Medical management of mild and moderate vesicoureteral reflux: followup studies of infants and young children. A preliminary report of the Southwest Pediatric Nephrology Study Group. J Urol 1992;148(5 Pt 2):1683–7.
5. Edwards D, Normand IC, Prescod N, et al. Disappearance of vesicoureteric reflux during long-term prophylaxis of urinary tract infection in children. Br Med J 1977;2(6082):285–8.
6. McLorie GA, McKenna PH, Jumper BM, et al. High grade vesicoureteral reflux: analysis of observational therapy. J Urol 1990;144(2 Pt 2):537–40.
7. Läckgren G, Wåhlin N, Sköldenberg E, et al. Endoscopic treatment of vesicoureteral reflux with dextranomer/hyaluronic acid copolymer is effective in either double ureters or a small kidney. J Urol 2003;170(4 Pt 2):1551–5.
8. Kirsch AJ, Perez-Brayfield M, Smith EA, et al. The modified sting procedure to correct vesicoureteral reflux: improved results with submucosal implantation within the intramural ureter. J Urol 2004;171(6 Pt 1):2413–6.
9. Puri P, Chertin B, Velayudham M, et al. Treatment of vesicoureteral reflux by endoscopic injection of dextranomer/hyaluronic Acid copolymer: preliminary results. J Urol 2003;170(4 Pt 2):1541–4.
10. Bisignani G, Decter RM. Voiding cystourethrography after uncomplicated ureteral reimplantation in children: is it necessary? J Urol 1997;158(3 Pt 2):1229–31.
11. El-Ghoneimi A, Odet E, Lamer S, et al. Cystography after the Cohen ureterovesical reimplantation: is it necessary at a training center? J Urol 1999;162(3 Pt 2):1201–2.

12. Ehrlich RM, Gershman A, Fuchs G. Laparoscopic vesicoureteroplasty in children: initial case reports. Urology 1994;43(2):255–61.

13. Atala A, Kavoussi LR, Goldstein DS, et al. Laparoscopic correction of vesicoureteral reflux. J Urol 1993;150(2 Pt 2):748–51.

14. Riquelme M, Lopez M, Landa S, et al. Laparoscopic extravesical ureteral reimplantation (LEVUR): a multicenter experience with 95 cases. Eur J Pediatr Surg 2013;23(2):143–7.

15. Smith RP, Oliver JL, Peters CA. Pediatric robotic extravesical ureteral reimplantation: comparison with open surgery. J Urol 2011;185(5):1876–81.

16. Akhavan A, Avery D, Lendvay TS. Robot-assisted extravesical ureteral reimplantation: outcomes and conclusions from 78 ureters. J Pediatr Urol 2014. [Epub ahead of print].

17. Hayashi Y, Mizuno K, Kurokawa S, et al. Extravesical robot-assisted laparoscopic ureteral reimplantation for vesicoureteral reflux: initial experience in Japan with the ureteral advancement technique. Int J Urol 2014;21(10):1016–21.

18. Schomburg JL, Haberman K, Willihnganz-Lawson KH, et al. Robot-assisted laparoscopic ureteral reimplantation: a single surgeon comparison to open surgery. J Pediatr Urol 2014. [Epub ahead of print].

19. Peters CA, Woo R. Intravesical robotically assisted bilateral ureteral reimplantation. J Endourol 2005; 19(6):618–21.

20. Marchini GS, Hong YK, Minnillo BJ, et al. Robotic assisted laparoscopic ureteral reimplantation in children: case matched comparative study with open surgical approach. J Urol 2011;185(5):1870–5.

21. David S, Kelly C, Poppas DP. Nerve sparing extravesical repair of bilateral vesicoureteral reflux: description of technique and evaluation of urinary retention. J Urol 2004;172(4 Pt 2):1617–20.

22. Casale P, Patel RP, Kolon TF. Nerve sparing robotic extravesical ureteral reimplantation. J Urol 2008; 179(5):1987–9.

23. Okamura K, Ono Y, Yamada Y, et al. Endoscopic trigonoplasty for primary vesico-ureteric reflux. Br J Urol 1995;75(3):390–4.

24. Gill IS, Ponsky LE, Desai M, et al. Laparoscopic cross-trigonal Cohen ureteroneocystostomy: novel technique. J Urol 2001;166(5):1811–4.

25. Yeung CK, Sihoe JD, Borzi PA. Endoscopic cross-trigonal ureteral reimplantation under carbon dioxide bladder insufflation: a novel technique. J Endourol 2005;19(3):295–9.

26. Kutikov A, Guzzo TJ, Canter DJ, et al. Initial experience with laparoscopic transvesical ureteral reimplantation at the Children's Hospital of Philadelphia. J Urol 2006;176(5):2222–5.

27. Canon SJ, Jayanthi VR, Patel AS. Vesicoscopic cross-trigonal ureteral reimplantation: a minimally invasive option for repair of vesicoureteral reflux. J Urol 2007;178(1):269–73.

28. Jayanthi V, Patel A. Vesicoscopic ureteral reimplantation: a minimally invasive technique for the definitive repair of vesicoureteral reflux. Adv Urol 2008;973616.

29. Valla JS, Steyaert H, Griffin SJ, et al. Transvesicoscopic Cohen ureteric reimplantation for vesicoureteral reflux in children: a single-centre 5-year experience. J Pediatr Urol 2009;5(6):466–71.

30. Patkowski D, Czernik J, Chrzan R, et al. Percutaneous internal ring suturing: a simple minimally invasive technique for inguinal hernia repair in children. J Laparoendosc Adv Surg Tech A 2006;16(5):513–7.

31. Chang C, Steinberg Z, Shah A, et al. Patient positioning and port placement for robot-assisted surgery. J Endourol 2014;28(6):631–8.

32. Health Quality Ontario. Robotic-assisted minimally invasive surgery for gynecologic and urologic oncology: an evidence-based analysis. Ont Health Technol Assess Ser 2010;10(27):1–118.

33. Parekh DJ, Messer J, Fitzgerald J, et al. Perioperative outcomes and oncologic efficacy from a pilot prospective randomized clinical trial of open versus robotic assisted radical cystectomy. J Urol 2013; 189(2):474–9.

34. Varda BK, Johnson EK, Clark C, et al. National trends of perioperative outcomes and costs for open, laparoscopic and robotic pediatric pyeloplasty. J Urol 2014;191(4):1090–5.

Minimally Invasive Techniques for Management of the Ureterocele and Ectopic Ureter
Upper Tract Versus Lower Tract Approach

Matthew D. Timberlake, MD*, Sean T. Corbett, MD

CrossMark

KEYWORDS

- Ureterocele • Ectopic ureter • Pyeloureteral duplication • Minimally invasive • Ureterocele incision
- Ipsilateral ureteroureterostomy • Heminephrectomy

KEY POINTS

- Evidence-based management for children with ureterocele and complete pyeloureteral duplication is not possible and treatment should be individualized.
- Management requires a tailored approach that involves consideration of renal function, severity of hydronephrosis and obstruction, drainage of the contralateral ureter and bladder outlet, and associated vesicoureteral reflux.
- Endoscopic decompression is best suited for (1) prompt decompression of ureteroceles in the setting of infection or obstruction, and (2) elective treatment of intravesical ureteroceles.
- For children with ectopic ureterocele undergoing heminephrectomy, the presence or absence of preoperative reflux is the key.
- Current data indicate that laparoscopic retroperitoneal heminephrectomy carries a higher risk of open conversion, significant urine leak, and innocent pole loss compared with a laparoscopic intraperitoneal approach.

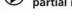 Videos of robotic-assisted laparoscopic ureteroureterostomy and robotic-assisted laparoscopic partial nephrectomy accompany this article at http://www.urologic.theclinics.com/

INTRODUCTION

A ureterocele is a congenital cystic dilatation of the intravesical ureter that may occur as an isolated anomaly, but most commonly affects the superior moiety (SM) of a complete pyeloureteral duplication (**Fig. 1**).[1] Classification of ureteroceles is shown in **Box 1**. Associated anatomic and pathophysiologic features (**Table 1**) include intravesical ureteral obstruction, dysplasia or obstructive nephropathy of the ureterocele-associated moiety (40%–70%), and vesicoureteral reflux (VUR) to the ipsilateral inferior moiety (IM) (50%) or contralateral renal unit (25%).[2] A tense ureterocele may mechanically obstruct the ipsilateral IM ureter, contralateral ureteral orifice, or bladder neck, although this is rare.

In the past, children with ureteroceles presented in early infancy with febrile urinary tract infection (UTI). Most cases are now discovered in the

University of Virginia Children's Hospital, University of Virginia, 118 Roy's Place, Charlottesville, VA 22902, USA
* Corresponding author. 118 Roy's Place, Charlottesville, VA 22902.
E-mail address: mdt4r@virginia.edu

Urol Clin N Am 42 (2015) 61–76
http://dx.doi.org/10.1016/j.ucl.2014.09.006
0094-0143/15/$ – see front matter © 2015 Elsevier Inc. All rights reserved.

urologic.theclinics.com

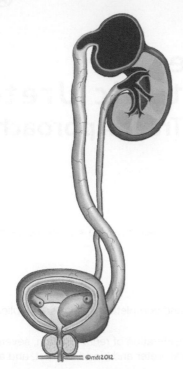

Fig. 1. Complete pyeloureteral duplication with upper moiety–associated ureterocele.

Table 1
Ureterocele classification and definitions

Intravesical	Cyst contained completely within bladder
Extravesical	Any portion extends into urethra or bladder neck
Cecoureterocele	Ureteral orifice in bladder, some tissue bulges beyond bladder neck
Ectopic	Orifice caudal to normal position of insertion on trigone
Stenotic	Small orifice
Sphincteric	Orifice within sphincter

antenatal or neonatal period during routine ultrasonography evaluation, and the natural history of patients diagnosed in the modern era is largely undefined.[3–6]

The goals of management for children with ureteroceles and pyeloureteral duplication (**Box 2**) are clear and include prevention of renal damage associated with obstruction or VUR and UTI, promotion of continence, and minimization of surgical morbidity.[7] However, the means of accomplishing these objectives remain a significant challenge in modern pediatric urology. Practice patterns are widely variable and no randomized controlled trials

exist to guide management decisions.[8] Selection of a treatment modality can therefore only be based on the balance between potential risks inherent to the condition and the summation of published results for a multitude of therapeutic alternatives.[3]

There is particular disagreement regarding the optimal management of patients with duplex system ureteroceles, especially in the presence of significant vesicoureteral reflux.[9–11] Current trends are away from single-stage open reconstruction (SM heminephrectomy, ureterocele excision, bladder base/neck reconstruction, and IM ureteral reimplantation) and toward conservative management and minimally invasive approaches.

This article discusses minimally invasive approaches for treatment of children with ureterocele and ectopic ureter. It addresses (1) nonoperative management before detailed discussion of (2) lower tract approaches (endoscopic ureterocele incision and ipsilateral ureteroureterostomy [IUU])

Box 1
Anatomic and pathophysiologic associations of ureteroceles

- Intravesical ureteral obstruction
- Dysplasia or obstructive nephropathy of the ureterocele-associated moiety (40%–70%)
- Vesicoureteral reflux (VUR) to the ipsilateral inferior moiety (IM) (50%) or contralateral renal unit (25%)
- Mechanical obstruction of the ipsilateral lower pole ureter, contralateral ureteral orifice, or bladder neck

Box 2
Goals of therapy for children with ureterocele and pyeloureteral duplication

- Prompt decompression of obstruction with infection
- Elimination of recurrent infection
- Relief of obstruction
- Elimination of clinically significant reflux
- Preservation of renal function (including functional moiety of a duplex system)
- Restoration and maintenance of continence
- Minimize surgical morbidity/minimize number of surgical procedures

and (3) upper tract approaches (ureterocele moiety heminephrectomy) in terms of selected operative techniques, patient selection, published outcomes, postoperative care, and follow-up.

CONSERVATIVE MANAGEMENT

The presence of ureterocele and duplication anomalies does not necessarily result in the development of clinically significant disease sequelae. Many investigators have begun to express concern about overtreatment and unnecessary surgery in this population. Several studies have shown that, if carefully selected, many asymptomatic children with ureteroceles can be safely managed initially without surgical intervention.

Shankar and colleagues[12] observed 52 consecutive patients for 15 years with nonobstructed IMs, absence of bladder outlet obstruction (BOO), nonfunctioning SMs, and less than grade III VUR. No patients underwent surgery or had UTIs at median follow-up of 8 years. Direnna and Leonard[13] similarly used a nonoperative approach in 6 patients without high-grade (III or IV) VUR, IM nonrefluxing hydroureteronephrosis, or BOO. Patients had either SM function less than 10% or greater than 10% with no obstruction. No patients developed UTIs or symptoms at 5-year follow-up. Hydronephrosis resolved in 4 of 6 patients and improved or remained stable in others, and VUR resolved in 4 of 6 patients and improved or remained stable in others.

Han and colleagues[14] showed that a nonoperative approach can be successful irrespective of ureterocele moiety functionality or presence of high-grade VUR given absence of high-grade obstruction on renal scan. They reported a series of 13 patients with either single-system ureterocele or complete pyeloureteral duplication in which 6 patients had good function in the ureterocele-associated moiety and 5 patients had ipsilateral grade III or IV VUR. All 5 patients with high-grade reflux had spontaneous resolution at 3-year to 4-year follow-up. Only 4 of 13 patients required surgical intervention for UTI or progressive dilatation. The investigators reported no significant difference between the nonoperative and operative groups with regard to hydronephrosis grade, reflux grade, or ureterocele size. Merguerian and colleagues[9] successfully observed a series of children with only minor SM dilatation and no evidence of obstruction on renal scan. None of these patients had experienced onset of symptoms or UTI at 5-year follow-up. Dilatation was stable in 6 patients and resolved in 4.[9]

Patients with multicystic dysplasia in the ureterocele moiety may also be candidates for observation given absence of ureteral dilatation, BOO, and high-grade reflux. Coplen and Austin[15] reported a series of 4 such patients, 3 of whom had associated grade I or II VUR. They noted ureterocele collapse in 2 of 4 (50%), resolution of VUR in 2 of 3 (67%), and spontaneous involution of multicystic dysplastic moieties in 4 of 4 (100%) by 18 months (**Box 3**).[15]

Current data suggest that a conservative approach is a favorable option for patients with small, asymptomatic, nonobstructive intravesical ureteroceles even if low-grade reflux is present. Patients with extravesical ureteroceles or multicystic dysplastic moieties may also be candidates in the absence of high-grade VUR or BOO. In any patient being managed conservatively, the development of BOO, symptomatic UTI, or significant worsening of upper tract obstruction should prompt consideration of operative intervention.

LOWER TRACT APPROACH: ENDOSCOPIC URETEROCELE INCISION

Endoscopic ureterocele decompression is a widely used, minimally invasive method of effectively achieving timely ureterocele decompression and decreasing the risk of UTI while avoiding extensive trigonal surgery in infants.[3,16–19] In recent years, endoscopic puncture has supplanted incision as the preferred technique.[20] Details of the procedure are shown in **Box 4**. In general, a larger incision offers more effective decompression with a potentially higher risk of de-novo VUR (**Fig. 2**).[3]

Alternative techniques include laser incision,[23,24] percutaneously assisted incision,[25] and concomitant ureterocele double puncture with intraureterocele fulguration.[26] Although initial data suggest success that is comparable with traditional puncture, outcomes likely reflect the anatomic and functional characteristics of the urinary system rather than the technique used.[25]

Box 3
Ideal candidates for a conservative management approach to ureteroceles

- Asymptomatic
- Good or absent function in ureterocele moiety
- Absence of grade III or IV VUR
- Absence of IM obstruction[a]
- Absence of BOO

[a] As shown by scintographic data or presence of marked nonrefluxing hydroureteronephrosis.

- Typically performed with an 8-Fr or 10-Fr endoscope and flexible 3-Fr monopolar wire electrode.
- The cutting current should be set high enough to ensure a clean puncture.[21]
- In older children, a pediatric resectoscope and Collins knife can also be used.[22]
- The bladder should be incompletely filled to achieve maximal ureterocele distension for incision. Incising distally on the ureterocele close to the bladder floor may prevent postoperative reflux.[22] For intravesical ureteroceles, the puncture can be low on the front of the ureterocele, allowing collapsed tissue to establish an antireflux valve.[16]
- For ectopic ureterocele, a single puncture of the intravesical portion of the ureterocele can be made just proximal to the bladder neck.[16]
- Decompression may be difficult to achieve if the Bugbee electrode displaces the inner mucosal coat of the ureterocele away from the outer layer.[16]

Patient Selection and Published Outcomes

Endoscopic puncture represents the treatment of choice for patients with ureterocele resulting in systemic infection, azotemia, or high-grade obstruction.[17]

In the elective setting, essential preoperative considerations include ureterocele type and position, upper tract anatomy, and presence of associated ipsilateral VUR. In the past, management has been based primarily on ureterocele position with endoscopic intervention preferred for intravesical ureteroceles, and upper tract approach or complete reconstruction used for ectopic, duplex system ureteroceles (**Boxes 5** and **6**).

This article next addresses (1) the general consensus that endoscopic puncture is an appropriate initial intervention for single-system intravesical ureteroceles.[5,17,21,27–29] This topic is followed by a review of more controversial applications of endoscopic intervention, including puncture as an initial intervention for children with (2) ectopic ureteroceles, (3) high-grade ipsilateral VUR, and (4) poorly functioning or nonfunctioning ureterocele-associated moieties.

Endoscopic Puncture for Single-system Intravesical Ureteroceles

Endoscopic puncture offers the greatest potential as a definitive treatment of patients with intravesical single-system ureteroceles. Successful decompression without reflux may be achieved in 70% to 80% of such cases.[20]

In a series of meta analyses, Byun and Merguerian[30] found a higher relative risk of reoperation after endoscopic management of ureteroceles that were (1) ectopic versus intravesical, (2) associated with duplex systems, and (3) associated with VUR preoperatively. The presence of multiple factors

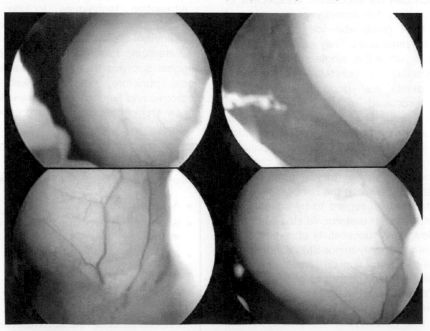

Fig. 2. Cystoscopic appearance of large intravesical ureterocele.

Box 5
Clinical scenarios in which endoscopic ureterocele puncture is traditionally used

- Obstructing ureterocele with systemic infection
- Obstructing ureterocele with severe nonrefluxing hydroureteronephrosis
- Intravesical ureterocele within a single nonrefluxing system

did not result in an additive effect on risk for reoperation. The investigators concluded that factors 1 to 3 represent proxies for trigonal anatomic distortion rather than independent risk factors for reoperation. This finding was subsequently corroborated by Di Renzo and colleagues[31] in a series of 45 patients undergoing transurethral puncture. Initial therapy was definitive in 24 of 45 patients (53%), whereas 21 (47%) required further surgery. Secondary surgery was more likely in the setting of duplex (58%) versus single system (18%), ectopic (61%) versus intravesical position (30%), and in the presence (61%) versus absence (37%) of preoperative VUR.

Endoscopic Puncture for Ectopic and Duplex System Ureteroceles

Ectopic position is associated with high reoperation rates after endoscopic incision. Husmann and colleagues[20] found that, in 28 patients with ectopic ureterocele undergoing endoscopic decompression, 18 (64%) required additional surgical treatment usually because of ipsilateral reflux.

Nonetheless, some investigators have begun to broaden their use of endoscopic puncture to include ectopic ureteroceles,[3] whereas others have combined endoscopic puncture with ureteral bulking agent injection in the setting of associated high-grade reflux (**Table 2**).[11]

Castagnetti and El-Ghoneimi[3] examined 41 neonates who underwent transurethral incision of

Box 6
Clinical factors associated with high reoperation rates following endoscopic puncture

- Ectopic ureterocele
- Duplex system
- High-grade preoperative VUR
- Postnatal diagnosis

duplex system ureteroceles within the first month of life. Twenty-four of 41 (58%) ureteroceles were ectopic. There was associated ipsilateral VUR in 13 (32%) and contralateral VUR in 7 (17%) patients. Endoscopic incision was an effective means of decompression in 40 of 41 patients. Ipsilateral VUR ceased in 6 of 13 ipsilateral IMs and 2 of 7 contralateral renal units. De-novo VUR in the punctured moiety developed in 13 of 41 cases (32%). Although 21 patients (51%) required secondary surgery (additional endoscopic procedure, reimplantation, or heminephrectomy) only 2 (5%) required surgery for de-novo reflux. There was no significant difference between intravesical and ectopic ureteroceles in the occurrence of VUR in the punctured moiety, rate of nonfunctioning SMs, or need for secondary surgery. The need for secondary surgery was significantly greater in patients with reflux before endoscopic incision.

Calisti and colleagues[11] applied an all-endoscopic approach in 46 patients with duplex systems associated with ureterocele and/or vesicoureteral reflux and examined the need for subsequent open surgery. After full diagnostic evaluation, patients underwent ureterocele puncture, bulking agent injection, or simultaneous puncture and injection. Indications to perform puncture included dilated upper system, recurrent UTI, or obstructive renographic pattern in a still functional renal moiety. Indications for ureteral bulking agent injection included patients with persistent grade 3 or greater VUR and recurrent UTI after antibiotic prophylaxis. Twenty extravesical ureteroceles and 13 intravesical ureteroceles were punctured. Twelve of 20 extravesical ureteroceles were associated with grade 3 or greater IM VUR, as were 11 of 13 extravesical ureteroceles. These patients underwent simultaneous ureterocele incision and bulking agent injection. Bulking agent injections alone were administered in 23 refluxing duplex renal units without associated ureterocele.

When the investigators applied puncture alone to duplex system ureteroceles, they observed successful ureterocele collapse in 9 of 10 (90%), secondary VUR in 5 of 10, and need for secondary surgery in 5 of 10 (50%) renal units.

When the investigators applied simultaneous puncture and ureteral bulking agent injection to duplex system ureteroceles with grade III VUR, they observed successful ureterocele collapse in 23 of 23 (100%), resolved or downgraded VUR in 11 of 23 (48%), secondary VUR in 8 of 23 (35%), and need for secondary surgery in 13 of 23 renal units (57%).

Overall, the all-endoscopic approach was successful and resolutive in 23 of 46 patients (50%)

Table 2
Endoscopic puncture of duplex system ureteroceles: preoperative, postoperative, and de-novo VUR

	Preoperative Ipsilateral VUR (%)	Resolved or Downgraded VUR (%)	De-novo VUR (%)	Secondary Surgery (%)
Castagnetti & El-Ghoneimi,[3] 2009, (N = 41)	32	18	32	51
Calisti et al,[11] 2011, (N = 46)	70[a]	63[a]	39	41

[a] Grade III or higher; patients received simultaneous puncture and bulking agent injection.

and significantly influenced by the grade of reflux. Seventeen of 46 patients (37%) subsequently required open ureteral reimplantation for persistent reflux associated with febrile UTI and 6 of 43 patients (13%) subsequently required partial or complete nephrectomy for severe renal dysplastic changes.

In the setting of ectopic ureterocele, transurethral puncture represents an effective short-term correction of upper pole obstruction but may not represent definitive therapy in most cases.[20,32] Many children require repeat puncture for adequate decompression or, more commonly, subsequent reconstructive surgery for persistent obstruction, recurrent infection, or persistent or de-novo reflux.[11,32] Furthermore, incision or puncture may increase the likelihood of future surgery in patients with no preoperative reflux, perhaps because of procedure-related de-novo reflux, although this remains unclear.[20,32] In light of these concerns, an upper tract approach has traditionally been used for ectopic ureteroceles.

Endoscopic Puncture in the Setting of Preoperative Vesicoureteral Reflux

There is some evidence to suggest that endoscopic puncture may be used irrespective of the presence of reflux, and that minimally invasive techniques may be used to treat children with VUR either inherent to a duplex system or resulting from previous endoscopic puncture.[33–35]

Adorisio and colleagues[36] applied endoscopic ureterocele puncture in 46 consecutive cases irrespective of the presence of reflux. Among 14 patients who had prepuncture VUR, 10 had spontaneous resolution in follow-up and the remaining 4 were corrected with endoscopic injection. Five of 46 patients developed de-novo reflux into the ipsilateral upper pole moiety. Two of these experienced spontaneous resolution, whereas 2 underwent endoscopic correction.

Calisti and colleagues[11] used bulking agent injection to refluxing duplex system ureters without ureterocele; they observed resolution or

improvement of VUR in 18 of 23 (78%) and need for secondary surgery in 5 of 23 renal units (22%). Perez-Brayfield and colleagues[33] similarly reported successful outcomes after endoscopic correction of complex ureterovesical anatomy in 72 patients, including 5 with VUR following ureterocele puncture or incision.

Endoscopic Puncture in the Setting of Poor or Absent Ureterocele Moiety Function

The risk of subsequent morbidity (eg, UTI, urolithiasis, hypertension, malignancy) conferred by leaving a nonfunctioning ureterocele-associated moiety in vivo is not well understood. Chertin and colleagues[6] examined the long-term morbidity associated with a nonfunctioning or poorly functioning moiety after endoscopic puncture in children with prenatal versus postnatal diagnosis. The groups had comparable percentages of intravesical and ectopic ureteroceles and nonfunctioning ureterocele-associated moieties. VUR was present in 23 of 35 of the prenatally diagnosed children (66%) and 12 of 13 (92%) of the postnatally diagnosed children. None of the prenatally diagnosed children had a postpuncture UTI, and they were less likely to require a secondary puncture or a secondary reflux procedure. Only 1 prenatally diagnosed child required subsequent heminephrectomy for high-grade reflux. These data suggest that nonfunctioning or poorly functioning renal moieties left in situ after endoscopic ureterocele decompression may not contribute to additional morbidity or frequently necessitate subsequent heminephrectomy. This possibility seems to be especially true in prenatally diagnosed children (**Table 3**).

Postoperative Care and Follow-up

Postoperative care and follow-up after endoscopic ureterocele incision is highly individualized. Hospitalization with intravenous antibiotics and monitoring may be necessary after acute decompression in the setting of systemic infection. In

Table 3
Prenatal versus postnatal diagnosis after endoscopic ureterocele puncture

	Median Age at Puncture	Preoperative UTI (%)	Postoperative UTI (%)	Secondary Puncture (%)	Secondary Reflux Procedure (%)	Heminephrectomy (%)
Prenatal diagnosis (N = 35)	4 mo	20	0	5	13[a]	3
Postnatal diagnosis (N = 13)	3.5 y	92	23	15	34[b]	15

[a] Endoscopic correction.
[b] Endoscopic correction in 2 cases, ureteral reimplantation in 2 cases.

the elective setting, it is frequently an outpatient procedure.

Postoperative imaging should include ultrasonography and voiding cystourethrogram (VCUG) at 4 to 6 weeks. Prophylactic antibiotics are often used until postoperative imaging is completed to assess for VUR.

LOWER TRACT APPROACH: IPSILATERAL URETEROURETEROSTOMY

IUU is an increasingly used alternative for children with pyeloureteral duplication in whom the obstructed moiety has significant functionality (**Box 7**).[37,38]

Conventional laparoscopic IUU is feasible and has been described.[39,40] However, the delicate intracorporeal suturing and fine reconstructive techniques necessary for the repair with current conventional laparoscopic instruments remains challenging for other than expert laparoscopic surgeons.[41] Several case series report successful robotic-assisted IUU procedures.[37,42–44] The authors prefer a robotic approach allowing superior visualization and more delicate tissue handing, as shown in **Box 8**.

Patient Selection and Published Outcomes

Overall clinical experience with minimally invasive IUU remains limited and published data describing outcomes and complications are sparse. Most

---

Box 7
Clinical scenarios in which IUU puncture is traditionally used

- Functional upper pole moiety
- No lower pole vesicoureteral reflux

---

investigators reserve IUU for children without IM VUR in order to avoid introducing reflux into a functional but anatomically abnormal upper pole moiety.[38,39,42] However, a few centers have begun using IUU for the management of duplex anomalies irrespective of the degree of ureteral dilatation, SM functionality, or presence of ipsilateral reflux (see **Box 7; Box 9**).[45,46]

Leavitt and colleagues[42] offered a series of 5 patients with a mean age of 61 months who underwent robotic-assisted laparoscopic IUU. All patients had complete pyeloureteral duplication with functional SMs confirmed with renal scan or magnetic resonance urography. No patients had VUR on preoperative VCUG. Mean operative time was 225 minutes, and mean hospital stay was 1.2 days. No complications were reported. All patients had resolution of presenting symptoms including UTI and incontinence, and all had significant reduction in SM hydronephrosis.

Gonzalez and Piaggio[40] performed 8 laparoscopic IUUs on 6 patients with complete ureteral duplication with preserved function of a refluxing or obstructing moiety. Two patients had reflux, which in both cases was confined to the IM. The investigators reported a mean operative duration of 257 minutes and mean blood loss of 2.7 mL. There were no intraoperative complications or conversions to open surgery. Mean morphine requirement was 0.13 mg/kg with a median hospital stay of 3 days. Two patients had febrile UTIs postoperatively. There was no significant hydronephrosis of involved moieties on postoperative ultrasonography.

After surgery, infection of the residual ureteral stump is a concern.[47] Lee and colleagues[48] found that 9 of 74 (12.2%) patients who underwent proximal ureteroureterostomy for duplex system anomalies required reoperation for complications related to infected residual ureteral

Box 8
Operative technique for robotic IUU

1. Cystoscopy and retrograde imaging is performed followed by:

   a. Catheterization of the recipient (ipsilateral nonobstructed) ureter

   b. The patient is repositioned to supine and slightly frog-legged, then secured in position. The robot is docked in modified side-docked, side-docked, or end-docked position near the foot of the table.

2. Three ports are placed. A camera port (8.5 mm or 12 mm) is placed through the umbilicus and 2 instrument ports (5 mm or 8 mm) are placed in the midclavicular line bilaterally 2 to 3 cm below the umbilicus. These ports can be moved more cephalad provide more room to operate intracorporally depending on the size of the child (**Fig. 3**).

3. The ureters are approached in a transperitoneal fashion and exposed by incising the peritoneum at the level of the iliac vessels.

   a. The ureters are mobilized 2 to 3 cm proximally and 2 to 3 cm distally.

   b. The recipient ureter is identified by the presence of the indwelling ureteral catheter and is mobilized from the donor ureter just caudal to the iliac vessels (Video 1).

   c. A hitch stitch is placed around the donor ureter.

   d. The dilated donor ureter is divided, and an effort is made to remove the distal ureteral stump of the dilated ureter to the deep pelvis as much as is feasible, minimizing manipulation of the lower pole ureter.

   e. Anteromedial ureterotomy of the recipient ureter is performed, followed by end-to-side anastomosis (Video 2).

   f. The lateral aspect of the anastomosis is accomplished first (Video 3) using the robotic instruments.

   g. A guide wire is fed through the recipient ureterotomy into the donor ureter and a double J stent is advanced to traverse the anastomosis.

   h. In addition, the medial portion of the anastomosis is completed. The double J stent is left indwelling (Video 4).

stump at a median follow-up of 5 years.[48] In these patients, larger preoperative SM ureteral diameter correlated with postoperative ureteral stump infections.

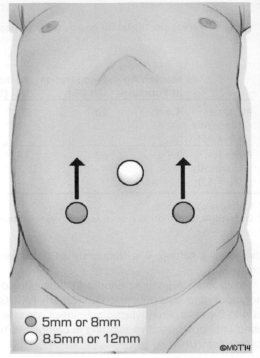

○ 5mm or 8mm
○ 8.5mm or 12mm

©MDT'14

Fig. 3. Port placement for robotic-assisted laparoscopic IUU. Arrows indicate cephalad port positioning for older children.

Ipsilateral Ureteroureterostomy in the Setting of Donor Ureteral Dilatation or Absent Upper Pole Function

McLeod and colleagues[45] performed IUU on 41 patients with ureterocele (17), ectopic duplex system ureters (25), and ureteral triplication (1) irrespective of ureteral diameter or SM function. Twelve of 41 patients were repaired laparoscopically, including 3 who required tapering of the donor ureter. The investigators reported 2 complications: 1 ureterovesical junction stricture unrelated to the anastomosis and presumed to be secondary to stent placement, and 1 anastomotic stricture in a child with massive ureteral dilatation requiring tapering. The investigators suspect that IUU is a safer, simpler procedure, and that it poses less risk to the innocent pole than SM

Box 9
Clinical factors that may discourage IUU

- Large donor ureteral diameter
- Significant recipient ureter VUR
- Systemic infections attributable to affected moiety
- Nonfunctioning affected moiety

heminephrectomy. They cite high reoperation rates after SM heminephrectomy for duplex anomalies.[49]

Chacko and colleagues[46] performed open IUU in 41 patients with dilated duplex system ureters. Thirty of these were in conjunction with ipsilateral ureteral reimplant of the common segment. Suboptimal outcomes included de-novo ipsilateral VUR requiring subsequent reimplantation in 2 patients, postoperative urinoma requiring drainage in 2 patients, persistent VUR in 3 patients, and ipsilateral urinary obstruction requiring percutaneous nephrostomy in 1 patient.

Superior Moiety Salvage Procedure Versus Heminephrectomy: Is the Upper Pole Worth Saving?

Some investigators have shown that SM salvage procedure (IUU, ureteropyelostomy) recoups only a modest percentile of overall renal function and may contribute to overall surgical morbidity in some patients. Vates and colleagues[50] retrospectively reviewed a series of 46 patients with unilateral obstructed SM of duplex system who underwent either SM salvage procedure (ureteropyelostomy, ureteroureterostomy) or SM partial nephrectomy. Three of 12 patients (25%) who underwent salvage procedure and 2 of 31 (8%) who underwent partial nephrectomy had symptomatic UTI postoperatively. Three of 12 patients (25%) required reoperation after salvage procedure compared with only 1 of 31 (4%) patients after partial nephrectomy. The average decrease in overall renal function among the 31 patients who underwent partial nephrectomy was only 2.25%.

Minimally invasive IUU can be an excellent option in carefully selected patients. However, the authors argue for judicious use in the setting of absent SM function, high-grade recipient ureteral VUR, and massively dilated donor ureter (**Table 4**).

Postoperative Care and Follow-up

On-the-table KUB (kidneys, ureter, bladder) may be obtained to confirm appropriate double J (DJ) stent position. If adjustment is necessary, repeat cystoscopy is performed. Patients are admitted the hospital for intravenous fluids and given ketorolac for postoperative pain control. The urethral catheter is removed on postoperative day 1. Patients are typically discharged on the afternoon of postoperative day 1.

The authors maintain patients on prophylactic antibiotics (most commonly trimethoprim-sulfamethoxazole 2 mg/kg/d, cephalexin 10 mg/kg/d, or nitrofurantoin 2 mg/kg/d) while the stent remains indwelling. Patients follow up (1) in 2 weeks for stent removal if a urethral string is left in place, or (2) in 4 to 6 weeks for cystoscopy and stent removal under anesthesia if the string on the stent was removed during the initial procedure. Renal ultrasonography is performed 6 to 8 weeks postoperatively.

UPPER TRACT APPROACH: HEMINEPHRECTOMY WITH PARTIAL URETERECTOMY

Upper tract approaches to pyeloureteral duplex system anomalies have traditionally included pyelopyelostomy, ureteropyelostomy, and SM heminephrectomy. The first 2 are seldom used because they seem to offer no advantage compared with SM heminephrectomy, and may portend a higher morbidity.[50]

With respect to heminephrectomy, laparoscopic retroperitoneal,[51–55] laparoscopic intraperitoneal,[56–60] robotic retroperitoneal,[61] and robotic intraperitoneal[62,63] approaches have been described.

Table 4
Complications associated with IUU in patients with pyeloureteral duplication

Complication	Epidemiology	Management Alternatives
Urine leak; urine extravasation	Suboptimal or disrupted anastomosis	Proactive stent placement, observation
Distal ureteral stricture	Aggressive ureterolysis or endourologic trauma	Percutaneous nephrostomy, endourologic evaluation and intervention
Persistent hydronephrosis	Clinically insignificant sequelae of previous obstruction vs persistent obstruction	Nuclear scan if suspicion for persistent obstruction
Anastomotic stricture	Aggressive tapering	Endourologic intervention, surgical revision, SM heminephrectomy
Recurrent stump infection	Reflux and stasis	Excision of stump

There are several advantages offered by these approaches compared with open surgery. First, the innocent pole is not directly manipulated as it often is in open surgery, which requires mobilization of the kidney from surrounding structures and downward traction for exposure. Such maneuvers risk torsion of the renal pedicle and consequent injury or thrombosis of innocent pole vasculature.[55] In contrast, a laparoscopic approach is performed with the kidney in situ with minimal traction on the pedicle.[52] This approach may reduce the risk of remnant pole vasospasm or vascular injury.[22] Furthermore, minimally invasive approaches offer a shorter hospital stay and improved cosmesis with comparable operative duration.[64]

Transperitoneal and retroperitoneal laparoscopic heminephrectomy are comparable with respect to operative duration, hospital stay, and analgesic requirements and both are superior to open surgery in these respects.[53,60,63]

The authors prefer a robotic intraperitoneal technique similar to that described by Lee and colleagues,[63] in part because of superior three-dimensional visualization and magnification afforded by the robot. This technique is described in **Box 10**. In our opinion, robotic technology allows more accurate distinction of the vascular and anatomic plane between upper and lower poles of the duplex system, as well as an improved ability to preserve innocent pole vasculature, parenchyma, and ureter.

Patient Selection and Published Outcomes

Heminephrectomy is appropriate for children with ectopic duplex system ureterocele without VUR and is definitive in 85% of such cases.[65,66] It may also be considered in the setting of cystic malformation of SM and nonfunctioning refluxing IM (**Boxes 11** and **12**).[63] Few long-term data exist with respect to long-term functional renal outcomes after minimally invasive SM heminephrectomy. Potential suboptimal outcomes include ipsilateral hemi pole functional loss, UTI caused by persistent VUR, de-novo VUR, and need for additional surgery.

Several studies have shown the utility of heminephrectomy, especially in children with absent SM function and absence of preoperative ipsilateral VUR. Selected case series reporting outcomes after minimally invasive heminephrectomy are discussed later, organized by surgical approach.

Laparoscopic Retroperitoneal Heminephrectomy

Jayram and colleagues[51] organized a multicenter review of 142 patients with median age of

---

Box 10
Operative technique for robotic-assisted laparoscopic heminephrectomy with partial ureterectomy

Patients first undergo.

1. Cystoscopy with retrograde pyeloureterogram to define the surgical anatomy. Ureteral catheterization is occasionally performed for intraoperative identification of the ureter draining the functional pole.

2. The patient is positioned in a 45° modified flank position.

   a. Three ports are placed. A camera port (8.5 mm or 12 mm) is placed near the umbilicus followed by insufflation of the abdomen. Two instrument ports (5 mm or 8 mm) are placed (**Fig. 4**). An additional 5-mm port for liver retraction can be placed in the right midclavicular line for left-sided cases.

   b. The robot is docked.

   c. The colon is reflected medially and both duplex system ureters are identified medial to the IM on the affected side.

3. In SM heminephrectomy, great care should be taken to avoid injury to the IM vasculature as it crosses anterior to the SM ureter (Video 5).

   a. The dilated nonfunctioning ureter is divided proximally allowing decompression of the dilated moiety. In SM heminephrectomy, the divided proximal SM ureter is passed beneath the IM vasculature (Video 6). The ureter is used to facilitate retraction and mobilization of the affected moiety.

   b. The demarcation between the functioning and nonfunctioning moieties is visualized and divided using hook cautery (Video 7).

   c. The SM ureter is dissected as far distally as possible and then divided. If the divided ureter is known to be refluxing, the stump can be oversewn with absorbable suture. If the ureter is nonrefluxing, the stump is left open (Video 8).

   d. The specimens are removed through the umbilical port incision.

11.4 months who underwent laparoscopic retroperitoneal heminephrectomy for duplex kidney. Eleven patients required conversion to open surgery. No major complications were described. Thirty-eight of 142 patients (26.8%) developed an asymptomatic renal cyst, 7 patients (4.9%) had a

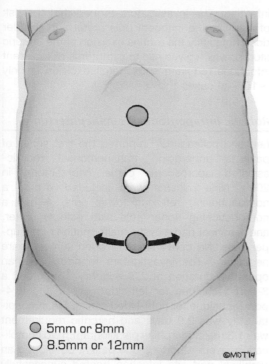

○ 5mm or 8mm
○ 8.5mm or 12mm

©MDT'14

Fig. 4. Port placement for robotic-assisted laparoscopic heminephrectomy.

postoperative urinoma, and 1 patient (<1%) required ureterectomy for UTI related to the ureteral stump of the excised moiety. Seven of 142 patients (4.9%) had renal atrophy or significant loss of function in the ipsilateral remaining moiety based on dimercaptosuccinic acid scan. Three of these patients required completion nephrectomy. Laparoscopic learning curve was not a factor in these cases because 6 of 7 procedures took place in the second half of the series. There was a higher rate of immediate postoperative complications (urinoma/hematoma, UTI), which was not statistically significant.

Valla and colleagues[52] published a series of 24 patients with a mean age of 22 months who underwent laparoscopic retroperitoneal heminephrectomy for pyeloureteral duplication. Mean operative duration was 2 hours and 40 minutes.

Box 11
Clinical scenarios in which heminephrectomy is traditionally used

• Nonfunctioning SM
• Recurrent infections attributable to poorly functioning SM
• Cystic malformation of SM and nonfunctioning refluxing IM

Box 12
Clinical factors that may discourage heminephrectomy

• Significant SM function
• High-grade preoperative VUR

Open conversion was required in 3 cases (12.5%). The investigators reported 9 intraoperative complications (37%) including 1 duodenal injury, 2 lower pole calycotomies, and 5 peritoneotomies. Mean hospital stay was 3.4 days. After surgery, 1 child had a large urinoma requiring percutaneous drainage and double J stent placement. There were no cases of lower pole atrophy or loss.

Lee and colleagues[53] reported a series of 14 patients undergoing laparoscopic retroperitoneal heminephrectomy, which was compared with an age-matched cohort of children undergoing open surgery. Operative time in the laparoscopic group was 194 minutes, compared with 193 minutes in the open group. No open conversions were necessary. The investigators reported a single urinoma in the laparoscopic group that did not require intervention. Laparoscopic patients had a mean hospitalization of 1.7 days compared with 4.7 days for the open group patients, which was significant. Postoperative narcotic requirements were also considerably less in the LRHN (laparoscopic retroperitoneal heminephrectomy) group and approached significance.

Wallis and colleagues offered a series of 22 patients with a mean age of 5 years who underwent laparoscopic retroperitoneal heminephrectomy for ureterocele (12), ectopic ureter (9), and VUR (5).[54] Four of 22 (18%) patients required open conversion because of inadequate exposure and were excluded. Three of 18 patients (17%) developed a urine leak managed with urethral catheter drainage and/or stent placement. Two young children in the series (aged 6 months and 7 months) developed functional loss of the innocent ipsilateral moiety confirmed by renal scan. One child presented with fever on postoperative day 3 and the other presented with hypertension 32 months postoperatively.

You and colleagues reported complete functional loss of the remnant pole in the only laparoscopic retroperitoneal nephrectomy in their series.[55]

Laparoscopic Intraperitoneal Heminephrectomy

Denes and colleagues[58] performed laparoscopic transperitoneal heminephrectomies in 17 patients with complete pyeloureteral duplication. Nineteen renal units were represented. Mean operative time was 147 minutes. No conversions to open surgery were necessary. Among 4 children with preoperative VUR, reflux resolved in 3 and improved in 4. Postoperative UTI was reported in 5 of 17 children (29%). The investigators reported development of empyema of the distal ureteral stump in 3 of 19 systems (15%).

Cabezali and colleagues[59] reviewed late outcomes and complications in 28 patients undergoing laparoscopic heminephrectomy. They reported manageable intraoperative bleeding in 3 patients (10.5%), urinomas in 2 patients (7%), a cyst at the resection margin in 6 patients (21.4%), hematoma in 1 patient (3.5%), and complete functional loss of the remaining pole (7%) caused by torsion of the remnant upper pole. The investigators concluded that extensive dissection and mobilization during heminephrectomy can lead to innocent moiety torsion after surgery.

You and colleagues[55] reviewed 17 children with complete pyeloureteral duplication with a mean age of 28 months who underwent laparoscopic heminephrectomy (15) and heminephroureterectomy (3) during a 5 and a half year period. The investigators reported a mean decrease in renal function of 2.8%. In intraperitoneal cases the only complication was prolonged urine leakage from a refluxing ureteral stump in 1 heminephroureterectomy. The investigators noted the presence of asymptomatic cystic structures in 6 patients.

In a series of 9 patients, Garcia-Aparicio and colleagues[57] reported a mean operative duration of 182 minutes with no open conversions and no complications, with mean hospital stay of 2.44 days.

In a series of 10 patients, Chertin and colleagues[60] reported an injury to the innocent pole ureter recognized intraoperatively and necessitating conversion to open surgery.

Robotic Retroperitoneal Heminephrectomy

Olsen and colleagues[61] reported on a series of 14 patients with a mean age of 4.9 years who underwent robotic-assisted retroperitoneal upper pole heminephrectomy during a 2-year period. The investigators reported a mean operative time of 176 minutes. Excluding 1 case, blood loss was less than 10 mL. Conversion to open surgery was necessary in 2 of 14 cases, as a consequence of uncontrolled bleeding in 1 case and lack of progression in another. One patient required further surgery to excise the distal remnant of the ureter because of recurrent infection. The investigators argued that the risk of injury to the innocent pole ureter and bladder does not justify the routine excision of the ureteric stump, which gives rise to symptoms or recurrent infections requiring subsequent excision in only ~10% of cases.[47,67]

Robotic Intraperitoneal Heminephrectomy

Lee and colleagues[63] reported the first series of patients undergoing transperitoneal robotic-assisted laparoscopic partial nephrectomy in 2009. Nine patients were included: 4 had a nonfunctioning refluxing lower pole, 4 had a nonfunctioning upper pole with ectopic ureter, and 1 patient had a cystic malformation of the upper pole. No conversions to open surgery were necessary. The investigators reported a mean operative duration of 275 minutes. They used a 3-port technique for left-sided cases and a 4-port technique for right-sided cases. Mean hospital stay was 2.9 days and narcotic requirement was 1.3 mg of morphine per kilogram. Two complications were reported. One patient developed an umbilical port site infection treated successfully with antibiotics. Another patient had an asymptomatic urinoma on postoperative ultrasonography that was drained percutaneously. The accumulation reaccumulated, but the patient remained asymptomatic and was observed. By 14 months, the collection had resolved. The investigators noted longer operative duration than is described for a pure laparoscopic approach, but linear regression analysis of operative time showed significant decrease in duration with experience.

Mason and colleagues[62] reported the largest series of children (N = 21) undergoing robotic intraperitoneal heminephrectomy to date. The investigators reported a 301-minute average operative duration using a 3-port technique in all cases. No conversions to open surgery were necessary. There were no intraoperative or postoperative complications in 18 of 21 patients, with a mean follow-up of 24 months. One patient had an anesthesia-related complication. One patient had extravasation of contrast during retrograde pyeloureterogram of the functional moiety that was concerning for iatrogenic forniceal rupture. This extravasation was managed with placement of a DJ ureteral stent, which was removed without incident 17 days later. One patient required reoperation for an incarcerated hernia of the 12-mm umbilical port site. Follow-up ultrasonography showed postoperative fluid collections in the bed of the excised nonfunctional moiety in 6 of 21 patients (29%). Two of the 6 resolved spontaneously

Table 5
Perioperative complications reported with minimally invasive heminephrectomy

All Follow-up Within 5 y	N	Open Conversion (%)	Significant Leak/ Urinoma (%)	Stump Infection (%)	Renal Loss (%)
Laparoscopic Retroperitoneal					
Valla et al,[52] 2003	24	3 (12.5)	3 (0)	0 (0)	0 (0)
Jayram et al,[51] 2011	142	11 (7.7)	7 (4.9)	1 (<1)	7 (4.9)
Lee et al,[53] 2005	14	0 (0)	1 (7.1)	0 (0)	0 (0)
Wallis et al,[54] 2006	22	4 (18.1)	3 (13.6)	0 (0)	2 (9.1)
You et al,[55] 2010	1	0 (0)	0 (0)	0 (0)	1 (100)
Total	203	18 (8.8)	14 (6.9)	1 (<1)	10 (4.9)
Laparoscopic Intraperitoneal					
Denes et al,[58] 2007	19	0 (0)	0 (0)	3 (15.7)	0 (0)
Cabezali et al,[59] 2013	28	0 (0)	2 (7.1)	0 (0)	2 (7.1)
You et al,[55] 2010	17	0 (0)	1 (5.8)	1 (5.8)	0 (0)
Garcia-Aparicio et al,[57] 2010	9	0 (0)	0 (0)	0 (0)	0 (0)
Chertin et al,[60] 2007	10	1 (10.0)	0 (0)	0 (0)	0 (0)
Total	83	0 (1.2)	3 (3.6)	4 (4.8)	2 (2.4)
Robotic Retroperitoneal					
Olsen & Jorgensen,[61] 2005	14	2 (14.2)	0 (0)	1 (7.1)	0 (0)
	14	2 (14.2)	0 (0)	1 (7.1)	0 (0)
Robotic Intraperitoneal					
Lee et al,[63] 2009	9	0 (0)	1 (11.1)	0 (0)	0 (0)
Mason et al,[62] 2014	21	0 (0)	0 (0)	0 (0)	0 (0)
Total	30	0 (0)	1 (3.3)	0 (0)	0 (0)

within 1 year, 1 decreased progressively but remained at 19 months, and 2 remained stable at 12 and 43 months of follow-up, respectively. A sixth patient was lost to follow-up after 3 months. All patients were asymptomatic. The investigators hypothesized that such collections may be prevented by formally closing the polar defect. However, most such collections can be reasonably followed and tend to resolve spontaneously with time (**Tables 5** and **6**).

However, heminephrectomy does not frequently represent a curative intervention for children with duplex system anomalies and VUR. Husmann and colleagues[20] found that in children with ectopic ureterocele in whom preoperative VCUG shows reflux, both endoscopic incision and heminephrectomy are definitive in only 16% of cases. Several studies have shown a prevalence of de-novo ipsilateral lower pole or contralateral reflux of 40% to 50% after upper tract surgery.[1,20]

Postoperative Care and Follow-up

Postoperative care is similar to is the care described earlier for IUU. Patients are admitted to the hospital for intravenous fluids. Ketorolac may be appropriate if hemostasis is favorable and renal

Table 6
Operative duration for alternate minimally invasive heminephrectomy approaches

Approach	Duration (min)
Laparoscopic Retroperitoneal	
Valla et al,[52] 2003	300
Jayram et al,[51] 2011	120
Lee et al,[53] 2005	194
Wallis et al,[54] 2006	174
You et al,[55] 2010	NR
Laparoscopic Intraperitoneal	
Denes et al,[58] 2007	147
Cabezali et al,[59] 2013	137
You et al,[55] 2010	167
Garcia-Aparicio et al,[57] 2010	182
Chertin et al,[60] 2007	NR
Robotic Retroperitoneal	
Olsen &Jorgensen,[61] 2005	176
Robotic Intraperitoneal	
Lee et al,[63] 2009	275
Mason et al,[62] 2014	300

Abbreviation: NR, not reported.
Data from Refs.[51–55,57–63]

function is normal. The urethral catheter is removed on postoperative day 1. Patients are typically discharged in the afternoon of postoperative day 1.

You and colleagues[55] cautioned that innocent moiety functional impairment caused by vasospasm or vascular injury might not be recognized and recommend postoperative nuclear scintigraphy in all patients. However, subjecting children to the invasiveness of radionucleotide imaging when asymptomatic with normal-appearing remnant renal moieties on renal ultrasonography may be unjustified.[62]

Some investigators recommend postoperative VCUG for patients with VUR detected preoperatively.[55]

SUMMARY

Evidence-based management for children with ureterocele and complete pyeloureteral duplication is not possible. Treatment should be individualized following consideration of renal function, severity of hydronephrosis and obstruction, drainage of the contralateral ureter and bladder outlet, and associated VUR and UTI. For children who warrant surgical intervention, early case series indicate favorable safety and efficacy data for several minimally invasive approaches. Practice trends and current research themes reflect a shift toward conservative and minimally invasive approaches. Future directions include defining the natural history of prenatally diagnosed ureteroceles, expanding case series data, and if possible prospectively comparing alternate minimally invasive techniques.

SUPPLEMENTARY DATA

Supplementary data related to this article can be found online at http://dx.doi.org/10.1016/j.ucl.2014.09.006.

REFERENCES

1. Coplen DE, Duckett JW. The modern approach to ureteroceles. J Urol 1995;153:166.
2. Merlini E, Lelli Chiesa P. Obstructive ureterocele - an ongoing challenge. World J Urol 2004;22(2):107–14.
3. Castagnetti M, El-Ghoneimi A. Management of duplex system ureteroceles in neonates and infants. Nat Rev Urol 2009;6:307.
4. Van Savage JG, Mesrobian HG. The impact of prenatal sonography on the morbidity and outcome of patients with renal duplication anomalies. J Urol 1995;153:768.
5. Upadhyay J, Bolduc S, Braga L, et al. Impact of prenatal diagnosis on the morbidity associated with ureterocele management. J Urol 2002;167:2560.
6. Chertin B, Rabinowitz R, Pollack A, et al. Does prenatal diagnosis influence the morbidity associated with left in situ nonfunctioning or poorly functioning renal moiety after endoscopic puncture of ureterocele? J Urol 2005;173:1349.
7. Pohl HG. Recent advances in the management of ureteroceles in infants and children: why less may be more. Curr Opin Urol 2011;21:322.
8. Merguerian PA, Taenzer A, Knoerlein K, et al. Variation in management of duplex system intravesical ureteroceles: a survey of pediatric urologists. J Urol 2010;184:1625.
9. Merguerian PA, Byun E, Chang B. Lower urinary tract reconstruction for duplicated renal units with ureterocele. Is excision of the ureterocele with reconstruction of the bladder base necessary? J Urol 2003;170:1510.
10. Afshar K, Papanikolaou F, Malek R, et al. Vesicoureteral reflux and complete ureteral duplication. Conservative or surgical management? J Urol 2005;173:1725.
11. Calisti A, Perrotta ML, Coletta R, et al. An all-endo approach to complete ureteral duplications complicated by ureterocele and/or vesicoureteral reflux: feasibility, limitations, and results. Int J Pediatr 2011;2011:103067.
12. Shankar KR, Vishwanath N, Rickwood AM. Outcome of patients with prenatally detected duplex system ureterocele; natural history of those managed expectantly. J Urol 2001;165:1226.
13. Direnna T, Leonard MP. Watchful waiting for prenatally detected ureteroceles. J Urol 2006;175:1493.
14. Han MY, Gibbons MD, Belman AB, et al. Indications for nonoperative management of ureteroceles. J Urol 2005;174:1652.
15. Coplen DE, Austin PF. Outcome analysis of prenatally detected ureteroceles associated with multicystic dysplasia. J Urol 2004;172:1637.
16. Hagg MJ, Mourachov PV, Snyder HM, et al. The modern endoscopic approach to ureterocele. J Urol 2000;163:940.
17. Cooper CS, Passerini-Glazel G, Hutcheson JC, et al. Long-term followup of endoscopic incision of ureteroceles: intravesical versus extravesical. J Urol 2000;164:1097.
18. Monfort G, Morisson G, Lacombe, et al. Simplified treatment of ureteroceles. Chir Pediatr 1985;26:26 [in French].
19. Singh SJ, Smith G. Effectiveness of primary endoscopic incision of ureteroceles. Pediatr Surg Int 2001;17:528.
20. Husmann D, Strand B, Ewalt D, et al. Management of ectopic ureterocele associated with renal duplication: a comparison of partial nephrectomy and endoscopic decompression. J Urol 1999;162:1406.
21. Blyth B, Passerini-Glazel G, Camuffo C, et al. Endoscopic incision of ureteroceles: intravesical versus ectopic. J Urol 1993;149:556.

22. Peters CA. Laparoscopy in pediatric urology. Curr Opin Urol 2004;14:67.

23. Marr L, Skoog SJ. Laser incision of ureterocele in the pediatric patient. J Urol 2002;167:280.

24. Jankowski JT, Palmer JS. Holmium: yttrium-aluminum-garnet laser puncture of ureteroceles in neonatal period. Urology 2006;68:179.

25. Ben Meir D, Silva CJ, Rao P, et al. Does the endoscopic technique of ureterocele incision matter? J Urol 2004;172:684.

26. Kajbafzadeh A, Salmasi AH, Payabvash S, et al. Evolution of endoscopic management of ectopic ureterocele: a new approach. J Urol 2007;177:1118.

27. Shekarriz B, Upadhyay J, Fleming P, et al. Long-term outcome based on the initial surgical approach to ureterocele. J Urol 1999;162:1072.

28. Jelloul L, Berger D, Frey P. Endoscopic management of ureteroceles in children. Eur Urol 1997; 32:321.

29. Coplen DE. Management of the neonatal ureterocele. Curr Urol Rep 2001;2:102.

30. Byun E, Merguerian PA. A meta-analysis of surgical practice patterns in the endoscopic management of ureteroceles. J Urol 1871;176:2006.

31. Di Renzo D, Ellsworth PI, Caldamone AA, et al. Transurethral puncture for ureterocele-which factors dictate outcomes? J Urol 2010;184:1620.

32. Jayanthi VR, Koff SA. Long-term outcome of transurethral puncture of ectopic ureteroceles: initial success and late problems. J Urol 1999;162:1077.

33. Perez-Brayfield M, Kirsch AJ, Hensle TW, et al. Endoscopic treatment with dextranomer/hyaluronic acid for complex cases of vesicoureteral reflux. J Urol 2004;172:1614.

34. Molitierno JA Jr, Scherz HC, Kirsch AJ. Endoscopic injection of dextranomer hyaluronic acid copolymer for the treatment of vesicoureteral reflux in duplex ureters. J Pediatr Urol 2008;4:372.

35. Lackgren G, Wahlin N, Skoldenberg E, et al. Endoscopic treatment of vesicoureteral reflux with dextranomer/hyaluronic acid copolymer is effective in either double ureters or a small kidney. J Urol 2003;170:1551.

36. Adorisio O, Elia A, Landi L, et al. Effectiveness of primary endoscopic incision in treatment of ectopic ureterocele associated with duplex system. Urology 2011;77:191.

37. Van Batavia JP, Casale P. Robotic surgery in pediatric urology. Curr Urol Rep 2014;15:402.

38. Prieto J, Ziada A, Baker L, et al. Ureteroureterostomy via inguinal incision for ectopic ureters and ureteroceles without ipsilateral lower pole reflux. J Urol 1844;181:2009.

39. Olguner M, Akgur FM, Turkmen MA, et al. Laparoscopic ureteroureterostomy in children with a duplex collecting system plus obstructed ureteral ectopia. J Pediatr Surg 2012;47:e27.

40. Gonzalez R, Piaggio L. Initial experience with laparoscopic ipsilateral ureteroureterostomy in infants and children for duplication anomalies of the urinary tract. J Urol 2007;177:2315.

41. Corbett ST, Burris MB, Herndon CD. Pediatric robotic-assisted laparoscopic ipsilateral ureteroureterostomy in a duplicated collecting system. J Pediatr Urol 2013;9:1239.e1.

42. Leavitt DA, Rambachan A, Haberman K, et al. Robot-assisted laparoscopic ipsilateral ureteroureterostomy for ectopic ureters in children: description of technique. J Endourol 2012;26:1279.

43. Traxel EJ, Minevich EA, Noh PH. A review: the application of minimally invasive surgery to pediatric urology: lower urinary tract reconstructive procedures. Urology 2010;76:115.

44. Thiel DD, Badger WJ, Winfield HN. Robot-assisted laparoscopic excision and ureteroureterostomy for congenital midureteral stricture. J Endourol 2008; 22:2667.

45. McLeod DJ, Alpert SA, Ural Z, et al. Ureteroureterostomy irrespective of ureteral size or upper pole function: a single center experience. J Pediatr Urol 2014. [Epub ahead of print].

46. Chacko JK, Koyle MA, Mingin GC, et al. Ipsilateral ureteroureterostomy in the surgical management of the severely dilated ureter in ureteral duplication. J Urol 2007;178:1689.

47. De Caluwe D, Chertin B, Puri P. Long-term outcome of the retained ureteral stump after lower pole heminephrectomy in duplex kidneys. Eur Urol 2002;42:63.

48. Lee YS, Hah YS, Kim MJ, et al. Factors associated with complications of the ureteral stump after proximal ureteroureterostomy. J Urol 1890;188:2012.

49. Banchieri FR, Grandinetti C. Ureterocele. Minerva Urol 1975;27:273 [in Italian].

50. Vates TS, Bukowski T, Triest J, et al. Is there a best alternative to treating the obstructed upper pole? J Urol 1996;156:744.

51. Jayram G, Roberts J, Hernandez A, et al. Outcomes and fate of the remnant moiety following laparoscopic heminephrectomy for duplex kidney: a multicenter review. J Pediatr Urol 2011;7:272.

52. Valla JS, Breaud J, Carfagna L, et al. Treatment of ureterocele on duplex ureter: upper pole nephrectomy by retroperitoneoscopy in children based on a series of 24 cases. Eur Urol 2003;43:426.

53. Lee RS, Retik AB, Borer JG, et al. Pediatric retroperitoneal laparoscopic partial nephrectomy: comparison with an age matched cohort of open surgery. J Urol 2005;174:708.

54. Wallis MC, Khoury AE, Lorenzo AJ, et al. Outcome analysis of retroperitoneal laparoscopic heminephrectomy in children. J Urol 2006;175:2277.

55. You D, Bang JK, Shim M, et al. Analysis of the late outcome of laparoscopic heminephrectomy in children with duplex kidneys. BJU Int 2010;106:250.

56. Wang DS, Bird VG, Cooper CS, et al. Laparoscopic upper-pole heminephrectomy for ectopic ureter: surgical technique. J Endourol 2003;17:469.

57. Garcia-Aparicio L, Krauel L, Tarrado X, et al. Heminephroureterectomy for duplex kidney: laparoscopy versus open surgery. J Pediatr Urol 2010;6:157.

58. Denes FT, Danilovic A, Srougi M. Outcome of laparoscopic upper-pole nephrectomy in children with duplex systems. J Endourol 2007;21:162.

59. Cabezali D, Maruszewski P, Lopez F, et al. Complications and late outcome in transperitoneal laparoscopic heminephrectomy for duplex kidney in children. J Endourol 2013;27:133.

60. Chertin B, Ben-Chaim J, Landau EH, et al. Pediatric transperitoneal laparoscopic partial nephrectomy: comparison with an age-matched group undergoing open surgery. Pediatr Surg Int 2007; 23:1233.

61. Olsen LH, Jorgensen TM. Robotically assisted retroperitoneoscopic heminephrectomy in children: initial clinical results. J Pediatr Urol 2005;1:101.

62. Mason MD, Anthony Herndon CD, Smith-Harrison LI, et al. Robotic-assisted partial nephrectomy in duplicated collecting systems in the pediatric population: techniques and outcomes. J Pediatr Urol 2014; 10:374.

63. Lee RS, Sethi AS, Passerotti CC, et al. Robot assisted laparoscopic partial nephrectomy: a viable and safe option in children. J Urol 2009;181:823.

64. Smaldone MC, Sweeney DD, Ost MC, et al. Laparoscopy in paediatric urology: present status. BJU Int 2007;100:143.

65. Husmann DA, Ewalt DH, Glenski WJ, et al. Ureterocele associated with ureteral duplication and a nonfunctioning upper pole segment: management by partial nephroureterectomy alone. J Urol 1995;154:723.

66. El-Ghoneimi A, Farhat W, Bolduc S, et al. Retroperitoneal laparoscopic vs open partial nephroureterectomy in children. BJU Int 2003;91:532.

67. Ade-Ajayi N, Wilcox DT, Duffy PG, et al. Upper pole heminephrectomy: is complete ureterectomy necessary? BJU Int 2001;88:77.

Management of the Bladder and Calyceal Diverticulum
Options in the Age of Minimally Invasive Surgery

Mesrur Selcuk Silay, MD, FEBU[a,b,c], Chester J. Koh, MD[a,b,c],*

KEYWORDS

- Bladder diverticulum • Calyceal diverticulum • Children • Minimally invasive surgery • Robotics
- Laparoscopy • Ureteroscopy

KEY POINTS

- Bladder diverticulum is a protrusion of the urothelial mucosa at a weak site of the muscular layers of the bladder.
- A calyceal diverticulum is a cavity within the renal parenchyma caused by narrowing of the forniceal or infundibular neck.
- Most of these entities are asymptomatic and may not require surgical intervention.
- If surgery is indicated, various minimally invasive treatment options including laparoscopy, robotic surgery, ureteroendoscopy, and percutaneous procedures have success rates at least equivalent to those of traditional open surgery in the pediatric population.
- Reduced morbidity, decreased hospital length of stay, improved cosmesis, and reduced pain medication requirements are potential advantages of the minimally invasive treatment modalities.

INTRODUCTION

Bladder and calyceal diverticula are rare clinical entities in children. Bladder diverticulum is defined as protrusion of the urothelial mucosa at a weak site of the muscular layers of the bladder, whereas calyceal diverticulum is a cavity within the renal parenchyma caused by narrowing of the forniceal or infundibular neck. The true incidence of both situations remains unclear because most of them are asymptomatic and may not require intervention. The estimated percentage of bladder diverticula

is approximately 1.7% of symptomatic children.[1] On the other hand, the incidence of calyceal diverticula was reported to be between 0.21% and 0.6% of in children who underwent intravenous urography.[2] In this review, these 2 different entities are discussed separately.

BLADDER DIVERTICULUM

There are 2 types of bladder diverticula in children: congenital (primary) and acquired (secondary). Although several theories for the congenital

Disclosure: The authors have nothing to disclose.
[a] Division of Pediatric Urology, Department of Surgery, Texas Children's Hospital, Baylor College of Medicine, Houston, TX, USA; [b] Scott Department of Urology, Baylor College of Medicine, Houston, TX, USA; [c] Clinical Care Center, Texas Children's Hospital, Baylor College of Medicine, Suite 620, 6701 Fannin Street, Houston, TX 77030, USA
* Corresponding author. Clinical Care Center, Texas Children's Hospital, Baylor College of Medicine, Suite 620, 6701 Fannin Street, Houston, TX 77030.
E-mail address: cxkoh@texaschildrens.org

Urol Clin N Am 42 (2015) 77–87
http://dx.doi.org/10.1016/j.ucl.2014.09.007

diverticula exist, the exact etiology still remains uncertain. One theory was proposed by Stephens[3] in 1979, who indicated that the diverticula occur because of "failure of muscle layer."[3] In that circumstance, either the complete absence or hypoplasia of detrusor muscle led to mucosal protrusion regardless of the normal voiding pressures. Garat and colleagues[4] examined the histologic appearance of the bladder diverticula in 7 children after surgical excision, and concluded that detrusor muscle fibers were present in all cases. Although the muscle fibers were histologically thin, these findings support the hypoplasia theory rather than the complete absence of the detrusor layer.

It has been reported that approximately 90% of congenital bladder diverticula are located adjacent to ureteral orifices.[5] These diverticula were first described by Hutch[6] in 1952 after his finding of a diverticula located superolaterally to the ureteral orifice. He also demonstrated the association of vesicoureteral reflux (VUR) and the diverticula in the same study. At present, diverticula in close proximity to the ureteral orifices are commonly referred to as Hutch diverticula in accord with this first description. The appearance of a Hutch diverticula is shown in **Fig. 1**. Previous reports have associated Hutch diverticula with VUR and varying degrees of renal dysplasia.[4,5] In addition, 10% of bladder diverticula can be located on the posterolateral wall of the bladder and are not associated with the ureteral orifices. These diverticula tend to be large and symptomatic, whereby children with posterolateral diverticula usually present with urinary stasis, retention, recurrent infections, and stone formation.

Secondary or acquired diverticula arise secondarily to high intravesical pressures of the bladder, which may be secondary to neurogenic diseases in children such as spina bifida. In addition, nonneurogenic diseases such as bladder outlet obstruction associated with posterior urethral valves (PUV) and urethral strictures can also lead to diverticula formation. Other causes may be iatrogenic as a result of previous bladder surgery.

Genetic predisposition and syndromic association of bladder diverticula have been described in the literature. Ehler-Danlos syndrome, Williams elfin facies, and Menkes kinky hair syndrome are some of the syndromes that may lead to higher risk for bladder diverticula in children.[7–9]

Most bladder diverticula are asymptomatic, small, and diagnosed incidentally during the clinical workup for urinary tract infections. The most common presentation in these children is recurrent urinary tract infections. Large diverticula may be associated with urinary stasis and incomplete emptying of the bladder,[10] which may lead to the urinary tract infections and bladder stones. Bladder diverticula may even present with pyelonephritis, whereby VUR was associated with the diverticula in a case report.[11] Lower urinary tract symptoms such as urinary frequency and nocturnal enuresis are other potential presenting symptoms, in addition to hematuria.[12] Although rarely seen, some children may present with urinary retention requiring clean intermittent catheterization.

Voiding cystoureterography (VCUG) is the gold-standard imaging method in the diagnosis of bladder diverticula. VCUG also provides additional information regarding the presence of VUR and the anatomy of the posterior urethra. Renal and bladder ultrasonography (US), computed tomography (CT), and intravenous pyelography (IVP) are other imaging modalities that may be helpful in diagnosing this rare clinical entity. In patients with affected upper urinary tracts, dimercaptosuccinic acid (DMSA) renal scan elucidates the differential function of the kidney and the presence of renal scarring.

Indications and Contraindications

The absolute indications for surgical management of bladder diverticula are still undetermined. For incidentally diagnosed asymptomatic small diverticula, close observation is an acceptable treatment option. As a general guideline, large

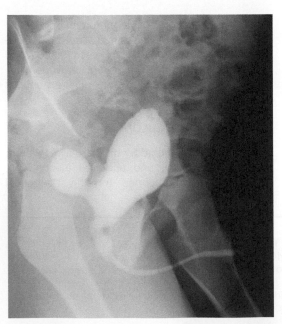

Fig. 1. Oblique appearance of a right-sided Hutch bladder diverticulum.

diverticula (>3 cm) are often surgically treated because these children are at higher risk for urinary tract infections, voiding difficulties, and stone formation.[1] At the time of the diverticula resection, antireflux surgery is also commonly performed. Bowel and bladder dysfunction should begin to be addressed preoperatively. One should keep in mind that the excision of bladder diverticula in children with hypotonic bladders may not resolve the lower urinary tract symptoms. For children with secondary bladder diverticula, it is essential that the primary cause, such as PUV, urethral strictures, or neurogenic bladders, should be treated concurrently.

Minimally Invasive Management of Bladder Diverticulum

Traditionally, open surgical repair by either intravesical or extravesical approaches have been the treatment of choice for bladder diverticula.[12,13] In the last 2 decades, with the advancement of the endourologic instruments, conventional laparoscopy, and robotic technology, there has been an increasing volume of reports on the minimally invasive management of bladder diverticula.[14,15] The main goal of these minimally invasive techniques are to achieve success rates similar to those of open surgery but with the typical benefits of laparoscopic and robotic surgery, such as shorter stays in hospital, improved cosmesis related to smaller incisions, and reduced pain medication. Although no prospective comparative trials for open and minimally invasive treatments have been performed to date for bladder diverticula, one can speculate that the improved cosmesis and shorter stays in hospital associated with minimally invasive approaches are desired if the high success rates associated with open surgery are maintained.

Current options for minimally invasive management of bladder diverticula are endoscopic resection, fulguration, endoscopic injection of bulking agents at the neck of the diverticula, conventional laparoscopy, and robot-assisted laparoscopic surgery.[14–18]

Technique

As endoscopic approaches (fulguration, injections, and so forth) have been reported elsewhere, this section focuses on laparoscopic and robotic treatment options for minimally invasive surgery for bladder diverticula in children.

The preoperative preparation and patient positioning for laparoscopic/robotic management are similar to those for other pelvic procedures such as ureteral reimplantation, orchiopexy, or bladder neck reconstruction.

Cystoscopy is strongly recommended to reveal enhanced anatomic information about the configuration of the orifices, location of the diverticula, and their associations. In addition, placing a ureteral catheter on the ipsilateral side may help to identify the ureter and the diverticulum during transperitoneal dissection for laparoscopy/robotic surgery. For the child with an extremely large posterior diverticulum, both ureters can be intubated to aid with identification. A urethral catheter is placed after prepping for bladder filling and emptying during the procedure. The patient is then positioned supine and secured to the table with tape in the Trendelenburg position to allow the intestinal contents to fall away from the pelvis. The robotic camera trocar is placed through an umbilical incision either via an open Hasson technique or with the aid of a Veress needle to create the pneumoperitoneum. The size of the camera trocar can be either 8.5 mm or 12 mm for robotic surgery, depending on the body mass index of the patient or surgeon preference. A 5- or 10-mm camera trocar can be used for conventional laparoscopy cases. Next, 2 robotic instrument ports (5 mm or 8 mm) are inserted along the axillary line at the same level of the umbilicus on each side. If a fourth accessory port is preferred by the surgeon, it can be inserted in the contralateral upper quadrant, where it can be used by the bedside assistant because it will be below the level of the robotic arms when the patient is in the Trendelenburg position. The configuration of the port placements is illustrated in **Fig. 2**. Following the completion of the port placements, the surgical robot (Intuitive Surgical, Sunnyvale, CA, USA) is docked from the foot position. For tall patients, the robot can be docked from the side of the legs to allow the patient to stay in the supine

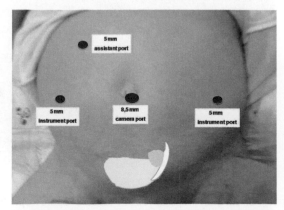

Fig. 2. The configuration of the port placement strategy for robotic-assisted laparoscopic bladder diverticulum excision. Note that the assistant port is optional.

position and avoid the dorsal lithotomy position and its risk for positioning injuries.

Once the camera, instrument, and assistant ports are placed, the bladder is filled with saline to visualize the bulge of the diverticulum. Afterward, a peritoneal window is created and the diverticulum is mobilized down to the diverticular neck. If the diverticulum is away from the ureter, the diverticulum is resected circumferentially using electrocautery or sharp dissection. The mucosal edges are closed using 4-0 absorbable sutures, and the muscle layers are approximated over the mucosal closure using 4-0 absorbable sutures. Alternatively, circumferential suturing can be performed at the neck of the diverticulum for the mucosal layer before resection of the diverticulum, similarly to an appendectomy.

If the ureter is in close proximity to the diverticulum, it is recommended to identify the ureter to prevent possible ureteral injury. If associated VUR on the ipsilateral side is present, extravesical ureteroneocystostomy can be carried out concurrently after diverticulum excision. The need for

ureteroneocystostomy should be decided individually according to the grade of the reflux, proximity of the diverticulum to the ureteral orifice, presence of kidney scarring, and the symptoms of the patient.

Finally the watertight anastomosis is checked by filling the bladder with saline, and the specimen is removed with the use of a laparoscopic pouch. A Foley catheter should stay in the bladder postoperatively for at least 24 hours, and placement of a Jackson-Pratt drain near the operational field is optional. The surgical steps of extravesical robotic-assisted laparoscopic bladder diverticulum excision are illustrated in **Fig. 3**.

Macejko and colleagues[19] previously reported that combination of flexible cystoscopy with robotic surgery for the illumination of the diverticulum may be helpful for diverticular identification and dissection during the extravesical approach. These investigators used this technique for 2 of their patients successfully, and concluded that this combination facilitates the surgical steps. Other investigators suggested the use of 1%

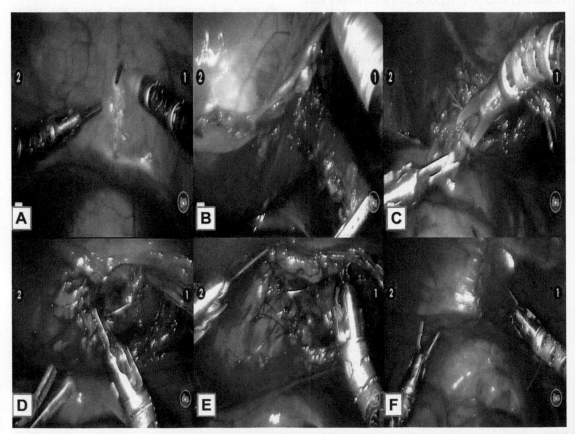

Fig. 3. Surgical steps of robotic-assisted laparoscopic bladder diverticulum excision. (*A*) Incision of the peritoneum overlying the bladder. (*B*) Mobilization of the bladder diverticulum by grasping the diverticula and dissecting down to the diverticular neck. (*C*) Excision of the diverticula after circumferential suturing of the neck. (*D, E*) Two-layer closure of the bladder detrusor layers. (*F*) Closure of the peritoneum overlying the bladder.

intravesical methylene blue during transperitoneal robotic excision of diverticulum.[20] Similar to the illumination technique, this offers assistance in the identification of the diverticular neck. Further studies are needed to establish its utility in children.

Alternatively, an intravesical pneumovesico-scopic approach with either laparoscopic or robotic-assisted diverticula excision can be performed in children. During this approach, after pneumovesicum is achieved, the diverticulum is retracted by grasping the mucosa of the diverticular wall intravesically. It is then dissected from the bladder completely, and the defect in the bladder wall is closed with 2 layers of sutures. Re-implantation of the ureter may also be necessary. The major limitation of this approach is the need for large enough bladder capacity of approximately 250 mL, which may not available in younger children.

Complications and management

Besides the general complications of laparoscopic surgery, one of the most common complications that may occur after laparoscopic/robotic bladder diverticula excision is urinary leakage, which may be secondary to incomplete closure of the bladder defect. A Foley catheter or suprapubic drainage may be helpful for spontaneous closure of the opening. Postoperative abscess formation can be seen, and should be treated with appropriate antibiotics or drainage if necessary. Ureteral injury, urinary obstruction, and hydronephrosis are other possible complications. If the diverticulum is close to the ureter, preoperative ipsilateral ureteral catheterization may help to avoid these injuries. Many of the ureteral complications may be conservatively treated by ureteral stent placement. Injury to other pelvic structures such as the vas deferens and rectum can be seen, especially in the small pelvic space of children.

Reporting, Follow-Up, and Clinical Implications

There is no standardized follow-up protocol after the minimally invasive treatment of bladder diverticula excision. In previously reported series, serial renal US and a postoperative VCUG at the 3- to 4-month mark are the most common imaging methods. It is important to address bowel and bladder dysfunction both preoperatively and post-operatively, as this may lead to urinary tract symptoms after surgery and may affect the surgical success rate. In addition, if clinical symptoms such as urinary urgency, frequency, and incontinence arise, anticholinergic therapy and urodynamic studies may be helpful in this setting.

Outcomes

Although the minimally invasive techniques for the treatment of bladder diverticula are increasingly becoming popular, publications regarding the pediatric population are limited to a few case reports. The initial reports for laparoscopic bladder diverticulectomy were published in1992 and included adult cases.[21,22] The first report of laparoscopic bladder diverticulectomy was published in 1994 in a 6-year-old boy who underwent simultaneous nephroureterectomy and diverticulectomy.[23] More recently, a pneumovesicoscopic approach was described by 2 different investigators.[24,25] Badawy and colleagues[24] reported 3 children with bladder diverticula who underwent pneumo-vesicoscopic diverticulectomy. The mean operative time was 133 minutes, and the patients were discharged home on the second day. Postoperative imaging confirmed the success of their procedures in all 3 cases. Other investigators[25] reported 6 children with a mean age of 5.6 years. The mean operative time was 110 minutes and no complications were encountered. Postoperative VCUG at 3 to 6 months after surgery confirmed the success of these procedures.

The first report of robotic-assisted bladder diverticulectomy in children was in 2009 by Meeks and colleagues,[26] who performed this procedure in a 12-year-old boy with a 12-cm diverticulum. More recently, Christmann and Casale[14] presented their experience with robotic diverticulectomy in 14 children. The mean patient age was 7.9 years and all children underwent a transperitoneal extravesical approach. The mean operative time including cystoscopy was 132 minutes, and most of the patients were discharged 1 day after surgery. All children were catheterized for 1 day. Postoperative urinoma or retention was not noted in any of the patients. The symptoms of the 6 patients who had diurnal enuresis preoperatively were all resolved within 3 months.

Current Controversies and Future Considerations

One of the controversies of bladder diverticula is the presence of VUR and its management. In earlier publications, it has been proposed that the presence of bladder diverticula decreases the spontaneous resolution of VUR in children. Therefore it has been recommended that uretero-neocystostomy should be carried out if surgery is planned for periureteral diverticula.[27] Reports with a different viewpoint have been published more recently. Afshar and colleagues[28] reported on 141 children with periureteral diverticula associated with various degrees of VUR, whereby they assessed the spontaneous resolution rates of these children in comparison with a control group consisting of 95 patients with primary VUR during a median follow-up of 47 months. In both groups the resolution, persistence, and the necessity of VUR correction rates were noted to be similar (diverticula patients: 43%, 27%, 30%, respectively; control patients: 44%, 31%, 25%, respectively). The investigators concluded that the natural history of VUR is similar in children with accompanying bladder diverticula, and therefore the treatment strategy for VUR patients with or without diverticula should remain the same.

Another controversy concerns the use of minimally invasive surgical approaches. The cumulative data in the literature reveals similar operative times and success rates for both intravesical and extravesical approaches.[14] Therefore, laparoscopic or robotic-assisted laparoscopic approaches remain as viable options for the treatment of bladder diverticula, and are subject to patient and surgeon preferences as well as the availability of the equipment. The advantages of robotic technology such as improved ergonomics for the surgeon, tremor cancellation, 3-dimensional visualization, and wrist-like movement do offer advantages over laparoscopy, and are especially helpful for reconstructive procedures of the bladder and ureter when suturing is used.

CALYCEAL DIVERTICULUM

Calyceal diverticulum is a cystic cavity within the renal parenchyma where the opening into this portion of the collecting system is associated with a thin forniceal or infundibular neck. It is lined by transitional epithelial cells that have no secretory function. However, urine can collect in these cavities by passive flow. Most of them communicate with other calyces, whereas others drain directly into the renal pelvis via a narrow isthmus. The retrograde pyelogram appearance of a lower pole calyceal diverticulum is shown in **Fig. 4**. The incidence of this rare entity is estimated at 0.3% in both children and adults.[29] There are several hypotheses for the occurrence of calyceal diverticula, but the exact etiology is still unknown. It may be acquired secondary to stone disease, infections, trauma, and VUR, or it may have a congenital origin. The embryogenic theory proposes that persistence of the branching of ureteral bud that fails to degenerate during metanephrosis may result in a calyceal diverticulum.[30] Approximately half of the calyceal diverticula are located in the upper pole, and this entity is more commonly seen in women than in men (63% vs 37%).[2] The size of the calyceal diverticula is usually less than

1 cm in diameter, although diameters of up to 7.5 cm have been reported.

Most calyceal diverticula are incidentally found, are asymptomatic, and usually do not require intervention. The natural history of this entity is as yet not well defined. Estrada and colleagues[31] retrospectively examined this entity in 22 children with a follow-up of up to 10 years. The mean age of the children was 5.4 years. Overall most calyceal diverticula remained asymptomatic, but 1 out of 5 had symptomatic enlargement. During the follow-up period, 43% underwent surgical intervention.

There are 2 types of calyceal diverticula, which are defined according to the communicating region. Type 1 calyceal diverticula communicate with minor calyces, whereas type 2 diverticula communicate with either the renal pelvis or a major calyx.[29] Another classification was proposed by Dretler[32] to assist in decision-making for surgery. In this system, types 1 and 2 were the calyceal diverticula with a short neck, type 3 diverticula had a long neck, and type 4 diverticula had an obliterated neck. Different treatment modalities including ureteroscopy and percutaneous management were recommended according to the classification algorithm.

The diagnosis of calyceal diverticula is often incidental after IVP or CT. US has a limited role unless the calyceal diverticulum is large or includes stones. Most diverticula remain asymptomatic but approximately 30% to 50% may present with several clinical presenting signs such as urinary tract infections, stone disease, flank pain, and

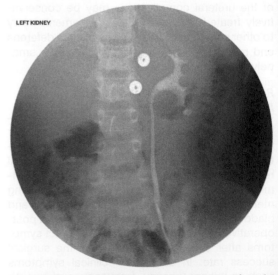

Fig. 4. Retrograde pyelographic appearance of a calyceal diverticulum within the lower portion of the left kidney.

hematuria. Calculi have been found in 9.5% to 39% of all calyceal diverticula.[33] Differential diagnoses include hydrocalyx, simple renal cysts, and papillary necrosis, as they have a similar appearance on diagnostic imaging. The association of calyceal diverticula with metabolic abnormalities has been proposed recently in cases where hypercalciuria and hyperuricosuria have been found in a limited number of patients. At least one metabolic abnormality was present in the series by Auge and colleagues[34] that included 37 patients, all of whom had stone disease associated with the calyceal diverticula.

Indications and Contraindications

The indications of surgery for children with calyceal diverticula are not well established. Expectant management is often used for small and asymptomatic diverticula, but surgery is warranted in children who have symptomatic enlargement of calyceal diverticula, symptomatic calculi, flank pain, abscess formation, recurrent upper urinary tract infections, and associated hematuria. In children with concomitant ipsilateral VUR, bladder procedures such as reimplantation should be considered.

Minimally Invasive Management of Calyceal Diverticulum

When surgery is indicated, there are several minimally invasive treatment options for the management of calyceal diverticula. The decision on the type of procedure usually depends on the location and size of the calyceal diverticula, presence of stone disease, length of the infundibular neck, availability of minimally invasive instrumentation, and surgeon and parent preference. Possible minimally invasive treatment options include ureterorenoscopy, laparoscopy, percutaneous ablation, percutaneous nephrolithotomy (PCNL), shockwave lithotripsy, partial nephrectomy, and marsupialization. Regardless of the treatment option used, the major goals of intervention are drainage or removal of the diverticulum, patency of the communicating channel, and/or removal of stones if present. The most common minimally invasive treatment options for calyceal diverticula are discussed here.

Technique

The most common treatment options for the management of calyceal diverticula are ureteroscopic, laparoscopic/robotic, and percutaneous approaches.

Ureterorenoscopy The preparation and positioning for ureteroscopic management of calyceal diverticula is similar to that for other ureteroscopic treatments in children. A negative urine culture should be obtained before the operation. Prophylactic antibiotics are administered intravenously in each case. Under general anesthesia, the procedure starts with routine cystoscopy in the dorsal lithotomy position on an endoscopy table that allows fluoroscopy guidance. After insertion of a hydrophilic guide wire into the renal collecting system, it is recommended to place a ureteral access sheath over the guide wire up to the renal pelvis so as to decrease the intrarenal pelvic pressure. If the ureter is too narrow to allow passage of an access sheath, a double-J ureteral stent can be left in place for 2 to 4 weeks for passive dilation. Once the access sheath has been placed, a 7.5F flexible ureteroscope and holmium-YAG laser can be used. Identification of the ostium is one of the crucial steps of the procedure, which can be performed with the use of contrast and fluoroscopy. After identification of the ostium, a guide wire is passed into the calyceal diverticula, after which a holmium-YAG laser can be used to incise the narrow infundibular neck. When the flexible ureteroscope reaches into the cavity, laser lithotripsy of the stone with extraction of the stone fragments is performed if present. Finally, the procedure is completed after the patency of the dilated infundibular neck has been confirmed. An indwelling ureteral stent is often left in place postoperatively for at least 1 week after the procedure.[33]

Laparoscopy/robotics The preparation and patient positioning for the laparoscopic or robotic-assisted laparoscopic management of calyceal diverticula is similar to that for other renal procedures such as pyeloplasty and nephrectomy in children. However, the authors recommend that the procedure begin with cystoscopy and retrograde pyelography while in the dorsal lithotomy position to ensure the location of the calyceal diverticula, and allow for placement of an open-ended ureteral catheter that will be secured to a urethral catheter. This action can aid in the identification of the diverticula with the injection of indigo carmine during laparoscopy.

After cystoscopic evaluation, the patient is positioned with the straight-arm technique.[35] When the patient is placed in the supine position, a large gel roll is used to elevate the patient's affected side lengthwise to obtain a 45° angle to the horizontal axis. After placing an axillary roll on the contralateral "down" side, the patient is secured to the table using wide silk tape. The table is then rotated to raise the ipsilateral side and allow the abdominal contents to fall away from the surgical area (**Fig. 5**). The authors use the straight-arm technique for both the laparoscopic and robotic-

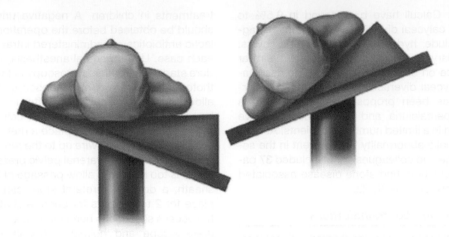

Fig. 5. Positioning of the patient using the straight-arm technique. (*From* Chandrasoma S, Kokorowski P, Peters CA, et al. Straight-arm positioning and port placement for pediatric robotic-assisted laparoscopic renal surgery. J Robot Surg 2010;4:29–32; with permission.)

assisted procedures in children. It is an alternative to flank positioning for kidney procedures. By maintaining the natural position of the child, the goal is to reduce the risk of unintentional sequelae such as upper extremity nerve palsy or positioning injuries.

After the ports have been placed, one proceeds with a transperitoneal approach. The camera port is placed at the umbilical site with either an open Hasson or Veress technique. After creation of the pneumoperitoneum two additional instrument ports are placed, one to the midline below the xiphoid process, the other to the ipsilateral lower quadrant on the midclavicular line. A fourth accessory port is optional, and is placed in the contralateral upper quadrant in the midclavicular line as shown in **Fig. 6**. The surgical robot is then docked for the robotic approach.

After mobilizing the colon and entering the perirenal space, the calyceal diverticulum can often be identified by the thin parenchyma at that site. If this is not visible, injection of indigo carmine through the previously placed ureteral catheter may assist in the identification by turning the color of the diverticulum surface to blue. If the calyceal diverticulum is still difficult to identify, a drop-in laparoscopic US probe can be used to identify the diverticulum location. Afterward, the parenchyma over the calyceal diverticulum is incised along the avascular plane with the use of electrocautery. Intradiverticular calculi are extracted if present, then the cavity is fulgurated until the infundibular neck is obliterated. If necessary, an absorbable suture can be used to ensure closure of the neck. The procedure is completed after placement of a Penrose drain near the surgical field.

Percutaneous treatment The percutaneous approach for the treatment of calyceal diverticula is another popular modality, especially if the child has a large stone burden inside the calyceal diverticulum. However, the success rates may be reduced if the cavity is small, which can render renal access as challenging. After ensuring the sterility of the urine by obtaining a negative culture, the patient is forwarded to the operating room. Prophylactic antibiotics are administered intravenously in each case. The procedure starts with routine cystoscopy and placement of an open-ended ureteral catheter while in the dorsal lithotomy position. Then the patient is repositioned to the prone position. After retrograde pyelography is performed, an 18-gauge percutaneous needle is placed directly into the calyceal

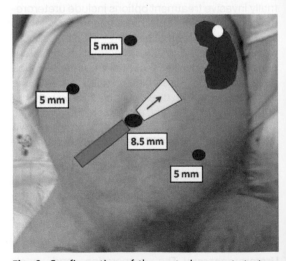

Fig. 6. Configuration of the port placement strategy for robotic-assisted laparoscopic calyceal diverticulum repair. Note that the assistant port is optional.

diverticulum for initial access. A safety guide wire is inserted and dilatation is sequentially performed under fluoroscopic guidance. Once the Amplatz sheath has been placed, a rigid nephroscope is used to visualize the collecting system of the diverticulum. If a calculus is present, it can be fragmented and completely removed from the cavity. Afterward, the cavity and the infundibular neck can be fulgurated with a holmium-YAG laser. A percutaneous nephrostomy tube inside the calyceal diverticulum is left in place at the end of the procedure.

Complications and management

Although ureteroscopic management of calyceal diverticula is generally a safe and minimally invasive procedure, complications are always a possibility. The most common complication is ureteral wall injury or perforation, which usually can be managed with an indwelling ureteral stent. In addition, various degrees of blood loss, ureteral avulsion, pain, and sepsis can be seen during and after the procedure. Although rare, major bleeding can be observed after infundibular neck incision, for which transfusion may be required in addition to placement of a percutaneous pigtail catheter. Laparoscopic complications are commonly associated with initial intra-abdominal access, where solid organ injury, bowel injury, and bleeding may be observed. In addition, if the infundibular neck is not completely obliterated, urinary extravasation can occur. Other potential complications can arise during percutaneous calyceal diverticula treatment that are similar to those associated with PCNL in children, such as bleeding or access-related complications including pneumothorax, bowel injury, and urinary extravasation.

Reporting, Follow-Up, and Clinical Implications

The most important parameter to monitor during the follow-up of children with calyceal diverticula is the clinical symptoms. One should keep in mind that most calyceal diverticula are asymptomatic and usually do not require surgical intervention. However, it is also important to regularly follow these patients to prevent possible sequelae associated with the diverticula. The follow-up for children with stones within the calyceal diverticulum is similar to the follow-up of other children with stone diseases. A metabolic evaluation may reveal important systemic abnormalities that may affect future treatment decisions. In children who have undergone surgical intervention, renal US and IVP can be used for follow-up radiographic imaging. If a stone is extracted, the stone analysis may be helpful for stone-prevention strategies. If a child presents postoperatively with fever and urinary symptoms, a urine culture should be performed to rule out urinary tract infection or sepsis. In addition, within the early postoperative period, urine extravasation may lead to flank pain and clinical signs of a urinary tract infection.

Outcomes

Most reported series concern the adult population, and the pediatric reports are often limited to small case series. Casale and colleagues[36] reported transperitoneal laparoscopic treatment of 3 children. All patients were symptomatic and had large calyceal diverticula. The mean operative time was 134 minutes, and the patients were discharged home on the second postoperative day. No complications were encountered during and after the surgery. The investigators concluded that laparoscopic management is a viable option, especially in children with type 2 calyceal diverticula and with thin overlying parenchyma. In another study by Estrada and colleagues,[31] the investigators performed 10 surgical procedures for calyceal diverticula in children. Of these, 6 underwent percutaneous ablation, 1 open marsupialization/ablation, 1 partial nephrectomy, and 2 laparoscopic ablations. After a mean follow-up of 3.1 years, no recurrences were observed. In one patient who underwent percutaneous ablation, the child presented postoperatively with flank pain, nausea, and vomiting 2 weeks after surgery. The investigations revealed a hematoma within the cavity, which was managed conservatively. The ureteroscopic treatment of calyceal diverticula with stone disease in adults revealed stone-free rates that varied between 19% and 94%. The symptom-free rate at follow-up of these patients also varied widely, between 35% and 100%.[2] Unfortunately, no reports on ureteroscopic management of pediatric calyceal diverticula exist in the literature. More studies are warranted to demonstrate the efficacy of such minimally invasive approaches for calyceal diverticula in children.

CURRENT CONTROVERSIES AND FUTURE CONSIDERATIONS

One of the most important controversies of calyceal diverticulum involves its diagnosis and necessary imaging. Simple renal cysts, hydrocalicosis, papillary necrosis, and renal tumors may appear similar to calyceal diverticula on diagnostic imaging. Therefore, careful preoperative evaluation and imaging that limits the radiation dosage to children is needed to ensure the correct diagnosis. With the development of finer minimally invasive instruments that are more suitable for use in the pediatric population, it is expected that the management of calyceal diverticula will continue to evolve toward minimally invasive approaches over time.

Another controversy is whether calyceal diverticula require surgical intervention. Close follow-up and assessment of the clinical symptoms and the associated abnormalities such as stone disease and VUR in these children will guide the clinical decision regarding surgical intervention. Because many of these children are asymptomatic, watchful waiting may be appropriate in most cases until bothersome symptoms arise.

SUMMARY

Both bladder and calyceal diverticula are rare entities in the pediatric population. Most of these are asymptomatic, detected incidentally, and often do not require surgical intervention. However, if surgery is indicated, with the advancement of pediatric laparoscopic and robotic instruments there are various minimally invasive treatment options currently available, which appear to have success rates comparable with those of traditional open surgeries. In addition, these minimally invasive options offer several advantages over open surgery such as minimal morbidity, decreased hospital length of stay, improved cosmesis, and reduced pain medication requirements. In sum, minimally invasive management of bladder and calyceal diverticula are viable options in the pediatric population.

REFERENCES

1. Psutka SP, Cendron M. Bladder diverticula in children. J Pediatr Urol 2013;9:129–38.
2. Waingankar N, Hayek S, Smith AD, et al. Calyceal diverticula: a comprehensive review. Rev Urol 2014;16:29–43.
3. Stephens FD. The vesicoureteral hiatus and para-ureteral diverticula. J Urol 1979;121:786–91.
4. Garat JM, Angerri O, Caffaratti J, et al. Primary congenital bladder diverticula in children. Urology 2007;70:984–8.
5. Tokunaka S, Koyanagi T, Matsuno T, et al. Paraureteral diverticula: clinical experience in 17 cases with associated renal dysmorphism. J Urol 1980; 124:791–6.
6. Hutch JA. Vesicoureteral reflux in the paraplegic: cause and correction. J Urol 1952;68:457–69.
7. Babbitt DP, Dobbs J, Boedecker DA. Multiple bladder diverticula in Williams "Elfin-Facies" syndrome. Pediatr Radiol 1979;8:29–31.
8. Daly WJ, Rabinovitch HH. Urologic abnormalities in Menkes' syndrome. J Urol 1981;126:262–4.
9. Levard G, Aigrain Y, Ferkadji L, et al. Urinary bladder diverticula and the Ehler Danlos syndrome in children. J Pediatr Surg 1989;24:1184–6.
10. Bhat A, Bothra R, Bhat MP, et al. Congenital bladder diverticulum presenting as bladder outlet obstruction in infants and children. J Pediatr Urol 2012;8: 348–53.
11. Rawat J, Rashid KA, Kanojia RP, et al. Diagnosis and management of congenital bladder diverticulum in infancy and childhood: experience with nine cases at a tertiary health center in a developing country. Int Urol Nephrol 2009;41:237–42.
12. Bogdanos J, Paleodimos I, Korakianitis G, et al. The large bladder diverticulum in children. J Pediatr Urol 2005;1:237–42.
13. Evangelidis A, Castle EP, Ostlie DJ, et al. Surgical management of primary bladder diverticula in children. J Pediatr Surg 2005;40:701–3.
14. Christman MS, Casale P. Robotic assisted bladder diverticulectomy in the pediatric population. J Endourol 2012;26:1296–300.
15. Eyraud R, Laydner H, Autorino R, et al. Robot-assisted laparoscopic bladder diverticulectomy. Curr Urol Rep 2013;14:46–51.
16. Orandi A. Transurethral fulguration of bladder diverticulum: new procedure. Urology 1977;10:30–2.
17. Clayman RV, Shahin S, Reddy P, et al. Transurethral treatment of bladder diverticula. Alternative to open diverticulectomy. Urology 1984;23(6):573–7.
18. Nadler RB, Pearle MS, McDougall EM, et al. Laparoscopic extraperitoneal bladder diverticulectomy: initial experience. Urology 1995;45:524–7.
19. Macejko AM, Viprakasit DP, Nadler RB. Cystoscope and robot-assisted bladder diverticulectomy. J Endourol 2008;22:2389–91.
20. Moore CR, Shirodkar SP, Avallone MA, et al. Intravesical methylene blue facilitates precise identification of the diverticular neck during robotic-assisted laparoscopic bladder diverticulectomy. J Laparoendosc Adv Surg Tech A 2012;22:492–5.
21. Das S. Laparoscopic removal of bladder diverticulum. J Urol 1992;148:1837–9.
22. Parra RO, Jones JP, Andrus CH, et al. Laparoscopic diverticulectomy: preliminary report of a new approach for the treatment of bladder diverticulum. J Urol 1992;148:1837–9.
23. Figenshau RS, Clayman RV, Kerbl K, et al. Laparoscopic nephroureterectomy in a child: initial case report. J Urol 1994;151:740–1.
24. Badawy H, Eid A, Hassouna M, et al. Pneumovesicoscopic diverticulectomy in children and adolescents: is open surgery still indicated? J Pediatr Urol 2008;4:146–9.
25. Marte A, Sabatino MD, Borrelli M, et al. Pneumovesicoscopic treatment of congenital bladder diverticula in children: our experience. J Laparoendosc Adv Surg Tech A 2010;20:87–90.
26. Meeks JJ, Hagerty JA, Lindgren BW. Pediatric robotic assisted laparoscopic bladder diverticulectomy. Urology 2009;73:299–301.

27. Barret DM, Malek RS, Kelalis PP. Observations on vesical diverticulum in childhood. J Urol 1976;116: 234–6.

28. Afshar K, Malek R, Bakhshi M, et al. Should the presence of congenital para-ureteral diverticulum affect the management of vesicoureteral reflux? J Urol 2005;174:1590–3.

29. Wulfsohn MA. Pyelocaliceal diverticula. J Urol 1980; 123:1.

30. Yow RM, Bunts RC. Calyceal diverticulum. J Urol 1955;73:663.

31. Estrada CR, Datta S, Schneck FX, et al. Caliceal diverticula in children: natural history and management. J Urol 2009;181:1306–11.

32. Dretler SP. A new useful endourologic classification of calyceal diverticula. J Endourol 1992;6(Suppl):81.

33. Canales B, Monga M. Surgical management of the calyceal diverticulum. Curr Opin Urol 2003;13:255–60.

34. Auge BK, Maloney ME, Mathias BJ, et al. Metabolic abnormalities associated with calyceal diverticular stones. BJU Int 2006;97:1053–6.

35. Chandrasoma S, Kokorowski P, Peters CA, et al. Straight-arm positioning and port placement for pediatric robotic-assisted laparoscopic renal surgery. J Robot Surg 2010;4:29–32.

36. Casale P, Grady RW, Feng WC, et al. The pediatric caliceal diverticulum: diagnosis and laparoscopic management. J Endourol 2004;18:668–71.

The Robotic-Assisted Laparoscopic Pyeloplasty
Gateway to Advanced Reconstruction

Gregory E. Tasian, MD, MSc, MSCE[a],*, Pasquale Casale, MD[b]

KEYWORDS

- Ureteropelvic junction obstruction • Minimally invasive surgery • Robotic pyeloplasty
- Urinary tract reconstruction

KEY POINTS

- Robotic pyeloplasty in children with ureteropelvic junction obstruction is safe and effective.
- Robotic approaches can be tailored to the size of the child and the anatomy of the pathology.
- Knowledge of the available instrumentation and the robotic platform is critical for successful repairs.
- Future studies are needed to assess the patient centered outcomes of robotic pyeloplasty in children.

INTRODUCTION

Historically, open pyeloplasty has been the standard treatment of congenital or acquired uretero-pelvic junction (UPJ) obstruction in adults and children, with overall success rates of 90% to 100%.[1–3] Although endopyelotomy[4,5] and retrograde dilation[6] are alternative methods of managing UPJ obstruction in children, the success of these two procedures is inferior to that reported for definitive surgical repair.[7] Advances in technology over the last 2 decades have led to the introduction of laparoscopic and robot-assisted laparoscopic pyeloplasty.

Kavoussi and Peters[8] and Schuessler and colleagues[9] independently reported the first successful laparoscopic pyeloplasty for adults with UPJ obstruction in 1993. With a success rate of more than 95%,[10] the magnification provided by laparoscopy improves visualization and control.

However, the operative times for conventional laparoscopic pyeloplasty are higher than open pyeloplasty in most series.[11,12] Additionally, laparoscopic suturing, particularly for children, is challenging and time consuming and has a steep and long learning curve because of its technical difficulty.

Robotic surgery mitigates many of the problems of conventional laparoscopy because of the precision of the movements of the robotic arms, ease in suturing, and 3-dimensional visualization. Consequently, robotic pyeloplasty may be easier to learn than conventional laparoscopic pyeloplasty.[13] Robotic pyeloplasty is now commonly performed for children with UPJ obstruction.[14]

INDICATIONS/CONTRAINDICATIONS

The robotic platform is a surgical tool that facilitates pyeloplasty and other reconstructive

a Division of Urology, Department of Surgery, Center for Pediatric Clinical Effectiveness, The Children's Hospital of Philadelphia, Perelman School of Medicine at the University of Pennsylvania, 3rd Floor, Wood Center, 34th Street and Civic Center Boulevard, Philadelphia, PA 19104, USA; b Department of Urology, Morgan Stanley Children's Hospital, Columbia University Medical Center, 3959 Broadway, 11th Floor, New York, NY 10032, USA
* Corresponding author.
E-mail address: TasianG@chop.edu

Urol Clin N Am 42 (2015) 89–97
http://dx.doi.org/10.1016/j.ucl.2014.09.008

urologic operations. The indications for robotic-assisted laparoscopic pyeloplasty are the same as those for an open pyeloplasty. These indications include

- Increasing hydronephrosis
- Progressive deterioration of renal function
- Recurrent urinary tract infection in the setting of obstruction
- Symptoms (pain, nausea/vomiting, hematuria)

Robotics increases operative efficiency compared with conventional laparoscopy and facilitates more complex reconstructive procedures, such as ureterocalicostomy for redo surgery as well as a primary modality for extreme cases of intrarenal collecting systems, which are covered later in this review.[15,16]

Although the indications for robotic pyeloplasty are the same as for open repair, the size and age of the child should be considered when using a robotic approach. When conventional laparoscopic pyeloplasty for children was first introduced, it was primarily performed on children older than 1 year, but improvements in instrumentation and surgeon experience have made laparoscopic pyeloplasty feasible in infants less than 6 months of age.[17] The robotic platform, which increases the range of motion and overcomes many limitations of laparoscopic surgery, has also been safely used to perform pyeloplasty in children 3 to 12 months old (6–11 kg).[18,19]

However, contraindications to robotic pyeloplasty exist (**Table 1**).

TECHNIQUE/PROCEDURE
Patient Positioning

After induction of general anesthesia, a regional anesthetic can be administered. The authors have found low-dose intrathecal morphine to be a safe and effective means of postoperative pain control.[20] An orogastric tube should be placed.

The authors do not place a stent before the pyeloplasty; but should one elect to do so, cystoscopy and stent placement can be done at this time. A Foley catheter is placed. The child is then positioned on the operating table in a modified flank position at a 45° to 60° angle with the affected kidney side up. A beanbag is used to support patients during the operation. The bed is flexed to create maximal separation of the distance between the iliac crest and inferior border of the 12th rib. An axillary roll customized to the size of the child is placed inferior to the contralateral axilla. The downside arm is positioned at a 90° angle to the body using an arm board. The ipsilateral arm is positioned in line with the body in a neutral position so that the anterior aspect of the arm is at the midaxillary line. The upper leg is fully extended and the lower is flexed at the knee. Gel pads are placed at all pressure points, and pillows are placed between the legs. Patients are secured to the table with tape applied below the knee, at or just below the hip, and just below the nipple line.

TECHNIQUE/PROCEDURE
Port Placement and Instrument Selection

A broad-spectrum intravenous antibiotic (eg, cefazolin) is given. Intraperitoneal access is obtained through the umbilicus using the technique with which the surgeon is most comfortable (eg, Hasson vs Veress needle). An 8.5-mm port is placed; pneumoperitoneum is obtained to a pressure of 10 mm Hg and a flow of 6 L/min. Laparoscopy is performed. Two 5-mm or 8-mm robotic ports are then placed. The superior trocar is placed in the midline between the umbilicus and the xiphoid. In infants, it may be necessary to place this trocar just inferior to the xiphoid. The inferior trocar is placed lateral to the rectus in the midclavicular line or more medial in small infants or in children with large renal pelves. Adjustment of port placement is necessary based on the anatomy of the UPJ and size of the child because of the smaller working environment compared with adolescents and adults. Although the pneumoperitoneum in adults will provide a 5- to 6-L working space, a 1-year-old boy will present a 1-L intra-abdominal space.[21] Consequently, the more limited working distance can restrict the mobility of the camera and instruments, and the chance of port site conflicts or trocar headpiece collisions is greater. Additionally, the thinner abdominal wall of children, especially infants, increases the probability that the trocar can be inadvertently dislodged. The authors limit the chance

Table 1
Contraindications to robotic pyeloplasty

Absolute Contraindications	Relative Contraindications
Untreated urinary tract infection	Prior intra-abdominal operations
	Small intrarenal pelvis (see "Difficult scenarios")
	Long ureteral stricture (see "Difficult scenarios")
	Small infant <6 kg

of this happening by anchoring the trocar to the abdominal wall with a heavy suture.[15] The robot is brought over the patients' chest and shoulder. The authors use a 0° lens, although the use of a 30° lens is an alternative option. A hook cautery is placed in the right arm, and a Maryland is placed in the left.

Mobilization of the Ureter and Pelvis

After medial reflection of the bowel, attention is turned to the kidney. A transmesenteric incision is usually possible for left pyeloplasties, and the colon often has to be reflected on the right. In transmesenteric approaches, a small incision is made in the mesentery of the colon near the UPJ taking care to avoid mesenteric vessels (**Fig. 1**). Blunt dissection with judicious use of hook cautery is used to expose the renal pelvis and ureter. The UPJ should be assessed for crossing vessels. Inevitably, a fibrous rind, which can be quite thick, is found around the UPJ. It is essential to remove this rind to facilitate anastomosis. The ureter should be freed from the rind but should not be skeletonized (**Fig. 2**).

Division of the Ureteropelvic Junction

Robotic Potts scissors are used for dismemberment (**Fig. 3**). For dismembered pyeloplasties, the ureter is spatulated laterally for about 1 to 2 cm (**Fig. 4**). Leaving the UPJ attached to the ureter allows one to use the UPJ as a handle and, thus, minimize handling of the ureter and aid in stabilization of the ureter during the spatulation. If so desired, a hitch-stitch passed through the abdominal wall just below the costal margin can be placed in the renal pelvis to expose and stabilize the UPJ (**Fig. 5**).

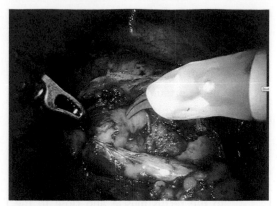

Fig. 2. Dissection of the fibrous rind around the UPJ obstruction.

Anastomosis

Large needle drivers or Black Diamond microneedle drivers are used for anastomosis. Depending on the size of the patient, the anastomosis is completed with a 6-0 or 5-0 poliglecaprone 25 suture on an RB-1 needle. The anastomosis is started at the apex of the ureteral spatulation, which is secured to the most dependent portion of the renal pelvis (**Fig. 6**). The posterior anastomosis is completed first using a running suture. Should a ureteral stent be placed, it can be done so at this time. The authors use a 14-gauge angiocatheter placed through the abdominal wall to direct a stent down the ureter. To do this, a guidewire is advanced beyond the distal end of the stent by 4 to 5 cm to decrease the likelihood of ureteral trauma (**Fig. 7**). At the beginning of the authors' experience, they filled the bladder with saline to which methylene blue had been added to allow reflux through the stent and, thus, confirm proper placement in the bladder; however, this is no longer routinely performed. The anterior anastomosis is then completed (**Fig. 8**).

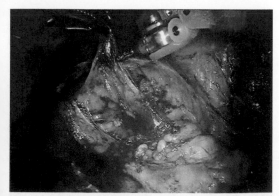

Fig. 1. A small incision is made in the mesentery of the colon near the UPJ taking care to avoid mesenteric vessels.

Critical instruments and supplies
• DaVinci surgical system
• 8.5-mm, 0° telescope
• Maryland bipolar forceps
• Monopolar hook device or curved scissors
• Robotic needle driver
• 8.5-mm trocar: camera port
• 5- or 8-mm trocars: working ports
• 5-0 or 6-0 monofilament absorbable suture

Critical operative steps

- Positioning: modified flank position with a 45° to 60° elevation of the flank
- Port placement
  1. Camera port: umbilicus
  2. Working port:

     Prepubertal/teenager: midline above the umbilicus and midclavicular line below the umbilicus

     Infant: upper port; subxyphoid in the midline/lower port; as lateral a possible to the rectus muscle and close to the inguinal region

- Docking: over the ipsilateral shoulder
- Approach: transperitoneal
- Access: transmesenteric on the left or by mobilizing the colon on the right
- Procedures: dismembered pyeloplasty versus modified Fenger plasty depending on the surgeon's experience or the presence of crossing vessel
- Step 1: UPJ obstruction exposure
- Step 2: incision of renal pelvis, UPJ, and ureter and spatulation of the ureter laterally
- Step 3: anastomosis using a running suture
- Step 4: if needed, a double pigtail stent placement in an antegrade fashion after the posterior closure is complete

DIFFICULT SCENARIOS
Intrarenal Pelvis

Because there is no extra pelvis, the ureter cannot be widely spatulated to increase the diameter of the anastomosis. In children without crossing vessels, particularly in the setting of a high-ureteral

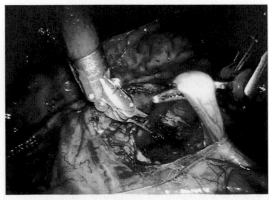

Fig. 3. Transection of the UPJ.

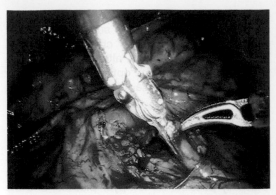

Fig. 4. Lateral spatulation of the ureter.

insertion, the authors favor a modified Fenger plasty. This technique obviates the tension that may result from the ureteropelvic anastomosis following dismemberment.

First, a longitudinal incision is made along the lateral aspect of the proximal ureter, carried through the UPJ and extended along the renal pelvis (**Fig. 9**). A 5-0 poliglecaprone 25 suture is placed at the apices of the ureteral and pelvis incisions to begin the transverse closure, which essentially results in a side-to-side ureteral-pelvic anastomosis (**Fig. 10**). The suture is then passed under the ureter to allow closure from the posterior aspect of the pelvis, running the suture toward the surgeon (**Fig. 11**). A stent can be placed at this time. The anterior anastomosis is then completed.

High Ureteral Insertion

The same principles apply to correct a UPJ obstruction caused by a high ureteral insertion. In such cases, the UPJ should be divided and the reanastomosis should be performed at the most inferior and medial aspect of the pelvis.

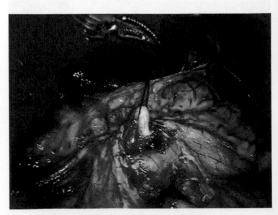

Fig. 5. Hitch stitch placed in the pelvis.

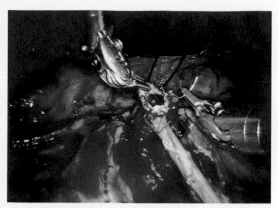

Fig. 6. Initial stitch placed through apex of ureteral spatulation to dependent portion of pelvis.

This procedure can be done by making an entirely separate incision or by extending the excision line laterally. An alternative approach is the modified Fenger plasty described above or a Foley Y-V plasty.

Long Ureteral Stricture

Culp-DeWeerd pyeloplasty

In rare cases when children have a long ureteral stricture associated with a UPJ obstruction and have a large extrarenal pelvis, a spiral Culp-DeWeerd pyeloplasty can be performed. In such a repair, a flap of pelvis, the base of which is oriented at the inferior-medial aspect of the posterior renal pelvis and the apex at the superior-lateral aspect. The flap is then rotated inferiorly to bridge the gap of the strictured area that needs to be excised. As this type of repair is only possible in patients with a large extrarenal pelvis and the working room in small children may be quite small, a Culp-DeWeerd repair may be technically difficult.

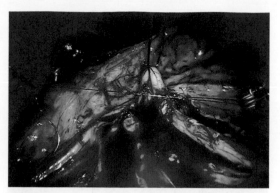

Fig. 8. Completion of anterior anastomosis.

Scardino-Prince pyeloplasty

An alternative repair is the Scardino-Prince vertical flap. The flap, which resembles a trap door, is composed entirely of the anterior renal pelvis, with the base of the flap at the inferior border of the renal pelvis and the lateral edge of the flap immediately above the UPJ. Care should be taken to ensure a wide flap base to ensure good perfusion of the flap and, therefore, reduce the probability of anastomotic stricture. Because the Scardino-Prince flap is based on the anterior pelvis, it allows for a more straightforward approach to a long proximal ureteral stricture using robotic assistance.

Ureterocalicostomy

Robotic-assisted ureterocalicostomy is an option in patients after failed pyeloplasty and a minimal pelvis, a long proximal ureteral stricture, or, rarely, for patients with a very intrarenal pelvis.[16] If the pelvis is not readily accessible, the authors think robotic ureterocalicostomy will be a better choice than redo robotic pyeloplasty. Unlike in straightforward pyeloplasties, reflecting the

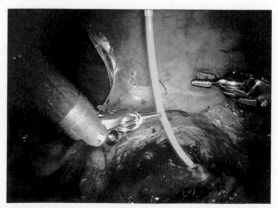

Fig. 7. Antegrade placement of ureteral stent over a guidewire.

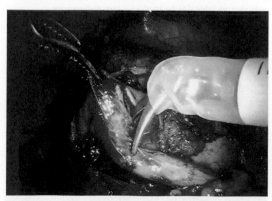

Fig. 9. Incision from renal pelvis through UPJ and along lateral aspect of the proximal ureter in a modified Fenger plasty repair.

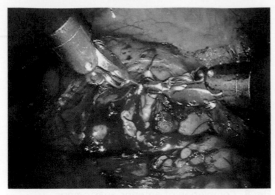

Fig. 10. Initiation of the transverse closure at the apices of the longitudinal incision.

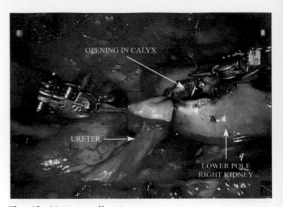

Fig. 12. Ureterocalicostomy.

colon is necessary. The ureter is transected at the level of the obstruction and then spatulated laterally. The parenchyma overlying the most dependent lower pole calix is amputated with hot scissors. Given the types of kidneys for which ureterocalicostomies are performed, there is usually minimal bleeding from the excision of the renal parenchyma. The posterior anastomosis is performed with a running 5-0 absorbable suture (**Fig. 12**). The authors routinely place stents for ureterocalicostomies using the same technique described earlier.

COMPLICATIONS

In a review of 5400 laparoscopic cases performed by 153 pediatric urologists, Peters[22] reported an overall complication rate of 5.4%. When excluding minor complications, such as preperitoneal insufflation, the incidence of complications decreased to 1.2%, of which 0.4% required additional surgical intervention. Peters also concluded that the greatest predictor of complication rate was surgeon laparoscopic experience. Complications of robotic pyeloplasty include the following:

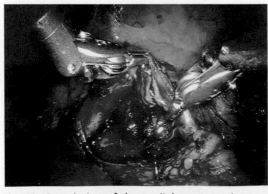

Fig. 11. Completion of the medial anastomosis.

- Bleeding: Usually coagulation and pressure is sufficient for control. Severe vascular injuries are rare and may require open conversion.
- Bowel injuries unrecognized at the time of surgery classically manifest at 2 to 3 days postoperatively as abdominal pain, particularly at the port sites, ileus, fever, and leukopenia. Clinical suspicion for bowel injury should remain high in this situation even days to weeks after discharge, as injuries caused by thermal may become apparent later because of delayed necrosis of the bowel wall. The surgeon should be cognizant of the proximity of the camera to the bowel, and thermal injuries can result from prolonged contact. Intraoperative injuries that are recognized at the time and are small in size can be repaired robotically by oversewing them if there has not been gross spillage of bowel contents. Otherwise, these necessitate open management.
- Ileus is not uncommon and typically resolves within 1 to 3 days.
- Wound infection should occur in less than 5% of cases and is managed by a 7- to 10-day course of antibiotics that cover common skin organisms.
- Hernia requires operative intervention.
  - Port site hernias may manifest as a bulge or tenderness at one of the port sites. If not definitive on physical examination, ultrasound can confirm a hernia.
  - Internal hernias are rare but could theoretically occur in a mesenteric defect.
- Thermal damage to tissues or organs is possible.
- Trocar or insufflation needle damage to viscera or vessels is possible.
- Persistent urine leak: Intra-abdominal urine leak usually results in severe ileus, which may include nausea and vomiting. Ensuring

Table 2
Outcomes

Study	Patients (n)	Mean/Median Age (Range) (y)	Mean/Median Operative Time (Range)	Mean/Median Hospital Stay (Range) (d)	Complications (n)	Success (%)
Atug et al,[26] 2005	7	13.0 (6–15)	184 (165–204)	1.2 (1.0–3.0)	1	100
Kutikov et al,[27] 2006	9	0.5 (0.3–0.7)	123	1.4	0	100
Lee et al,[28] 2006	33	7.9 (0.2–19.6)	219 (133–401)	2.3 (0.5–6.0)	1	93.9
Yee et al,[29] 2006	8	11.5 (6.4–15.6)	363 (255–522)	2.4 (1.0–5.0)	1	100
Olsen et al,[30] 2007	67	7.9 (1.7–17.1)	143 (93–300)	2.0 (1.0–6.0)	12	94
Franco et al,[31] 2007	15	11.9 (4.0–18.0)	223 (150–290)	Not reported	4	Not reported
Freilich et al,[32] 2008	5	9.5 (3.4–14.0)	384 (285–541)	2.4 (1.3–3.6)	0	100
Chan et al,[33] 2010	5	—	219 (105–420)	—	0	100

Data from Refs.[26–33]

proper stent placement, or placing a stent if one was not placed intraoperatively, is necessary. Draining the bladder through a Foley catheter often helps facilitate resolution of the leak if a stent alone does not resolve the leak.

- Stent migration: Depending on when the stent migrates after the pyeloplasty, either removing or replacing the stent is necessary.
- Urinary tract infection: Postoperative urinary infections should be managed with 10 to 14 days of antibiotics. If signs of sepsis continue despite proper urinary drainage and antibiotics, an abscess or infected urinoma should be assessed with an ultrasound and/or computed tomography scan.
- Reobstruction (<5%): Although rare, reobstruction presents a difficult problem, particularly if the pelvis was reduced on the initial pyeloplasty. In ureteral strictures less than 10 mm and in children older than 4 years, retrograde dilation with stenting may be considered,[23] although success is lower than with redo pyeloplasty. Redo robotic pyeloplasty is usually successful and can address the spectrum of causes responsible for initial pyeloplasty failure, including missed crossing vessels, ureteral stricture, and periureteral fibrosis.[24]

POSTOPERATIVE CARE

Most children spend one night in the hospital. Diet is begun immediately and advanced as tolerated. If the child is eating well, the Foley catheter is removed on the first postoperative day. If a stent was placed, it can be removed in 4 to 6 weeks. The optimal surveillance imaging protocol after pyeloplasty has not been defined. Recently, Romao and colleagues[25] demonstrated that no patients in whom the anterior-posterior diameter of the renal pelvis decreased by at least 38% developed recurrent obstruction. This finding suggests that ultrasound may be an effective screening tool to identify patients who are at a low risk for recurrent obstruction and, thus, may not need postoperative functional imaging.

The reported studies in **Table 2** are limited by their retrospective design, differences in age, dissimilar definitions of complications and outcomes, systematic differences in patient selection (bilateral UPJ obstruction[32]) and operative approach (eg, retroperitoneal[30]), and lengths of follow-up time over which success was determined. Despite these differences, the success of robotic pyeloplasty is consistently high.

CURRENT CONTROVERSIES/FUTURE CONSIDERATIONS

To date, no studies have assessed the cost-effectiveness of robotic versus open pyeloplasty in children. Such studies would allow for an appreciation of the costs associated with the presumed benefits of robotic surgery, including cosmesis, pain, and length of stay or convalescence. In addition to the fixed costs of the robotic platform, the costs of the increase operative time that must be overcome before a surgeon achieving proficiency should be considered. For example, the costs associated with becoming proficient in robotic prostatectomy were estimated to be more than $200,000.[34] Discussion about and studies on ways to increase the efficiency and decrease the costs of overcoming the learning curve for robotic pyeloplasty while maintaining excellent surgical outcomes are necessary. It is possible that surgical simulation could help achieve these goals, particularly in training programs given the association between operative volume and increasing facility with robotic pyeloplasty.[35–37] Finally, given the challenges of identifying universally accepted and objective outcomes for reconstructive surgery in general and robotic pyeloplasty, specifically, more work is needed to define the clinically important patient-reported outcomes, such as time off school/work as well as operative success.

SUMMARY

Robotic pyeloplasty is now a standard approach for children with UPJ obstruction that is safe and has success rates similar to open pyeloplasty. Understanding the fundamentals of robotic surgery and patient anatomy allows adaptation of robotic pyeloplasty for difficult cases for which standard dismembered pyeloplasty may not be optimal.

REFERENCES

1. Brooks JD, Kavoussi LR, Preminger GM, et al. Comparison of open and endourologic approaches to the obstructed ureteropelvic junction. Urology 1995;46:791–5.
2. Notley RG, Beaugie JM. The long-term follow-up of Anderson-Hynes pyeloplasty for hydronephrosis. Br J Urol 1973;45:464–7.
3. Persky L, Krause JR, Boltuch RL. Initial complications and late results in dismembered pyeloplasty. J Urol 1977;118:162–5.
4. Motola JA, Badlani GH, Smith AD. Results of 212 consecutive endopyelotomies: an 8-year followup. J Urol 1993;149:453–6.

5. Tan HL, Najmaldin A, Webb DR. Endopyelotomy for pelvi-ureteric junction obstruction in children. Eur Urol 1993;24:84–8.

6. Tan HL, Roberts JP, Grattan-Smith D. Retrograde balloon dilation of ureteropelvic obstructions in infants and children: early results. Urology 1995;46:89–91.

7. Ahmed S, Crankson S, Sripathi V. Pelviureteric obstruction in children: conventional pyeloplasty is superior to endo-urology. Aust N Z J Surg 1998;68: 641–2.

8. Kavoussi LR, Peters CA. Laparoscopic pyeloplasty. J Urol 1993;150:1891–4.

9. Schuessler WW, Grune MT, Tecuanhuey LV, et al. Laparoscopic dismembered pyeloplasty. J Urol 1993;150:1795–9.

10. Ben Slama MR, Salomon L, Hoznek A, et al. Extraperitoneal laparoscopic repair of ureteropelvic junction obstruction: initial experience in 15 cases. Urology 2000;56:45–8.

11. Piaggio LA, Franc-Guimond J, Noh PH, et al. Transperitoneal laparoscopic pyeloplasty for primary repair of ureteropelvic junction obstruction in infants and children: comparison with open surgery. J Urol 2007;178:1579–83.

12. Ravish IR, Nerli RB, Reddy MN, et al. Laparoscopic pyeloplasty compared with open pyeloplasty in children. J Endourol 2007;21:897–902.

13. Peters C. Laparoscopy in paediatric urology: adoption of innovative technology. BJU Int 2003; 92(Suppl 1):52–7.

14. Varda BK, Johnson EK, Clark C, et al. National trends of perioperative outcomes and costs for open, laparoscopic and robotic pediatric pyeloplasty. J Urol 2014;191:1090–5.

15. Casale P. Robotic pediatric urology. Expert Rev Med Devices 2008;5:59–64.

16. Casale P, Mucksavage P, Resnick M, et al. Robotic ureterocalicostomy in the pediatric population. J Urol 2008;180:2643–8.

17. Kutikov A, Resnick M, Casale P. Laparoscopic pyeloplasty in the infant younger than 6 months–is it technically possible? J Urol 2006;175:1477–9 [discussion: 1479].

18. Bansal D, Cost NG, Bean CM, et al. Infant robotassisted laparoscopic upper urinary tract reconstructive surgery. J Pediatr Urol 2014. [Epub ahead of print].

19. Bansal D, Cost NG, DeFoor WR Jr, et al. Infant robotic pyeloplasty: comparison with an open cohort. J Pediatr Urol 2014;10:380–5.

20. Ganesh A, Kim A, Casale P, et al. Low-dose intrathecal morphine for postoperative analgesia in children. Anesth Analg 2007;104:271–6.

21. Kutikov A, Fossett LK, Ramchandani P, et al. Incidence of benign pathologic findings at partial nephrectomy for solitary renal mass presumed to be renal cell carcinoma on preoperative imaging. Urology 2006;68:737–40.

22. Peters CA. Complications in pediatric urological laparoscopy: results of a survey. J Urol 1996;155:1070–3.

23. Braga LH, Lorenzo AJ, Skeldon S, et al. Failed pyeloplasty in children: comparative analysis of retrograde endopyelotomy versus redo pyeloplasty. J Urol 2007;178:2571–5 [discussion: 2575].

24. Hemal AK, Mishra S, Mukharjee S, et al. Robot assisted laparoscopic pyeloplasty in patients of ureteropelvic junction obstruction with previously failed open surgical repair. Int J Urol 2008;15:744–6.

25. Romao RL, Farhat WA, Pippi Salle JL, et al. Early postoperative ultrasound after open pyeloplasty in children with prenatal hydronephrosis helps identify low risk of recurrent obstruction. J Urol 2012;188:2347–53.

26. Atug F, Woods M, Burgess SV, et al. Robotic assisted laparoscopic pyeloplasty in children. J Urol 2005;174:1440–2.

27. Kutikov A, Nguyen M, Guzzo T, et al. Robot assisted pyeloplasty in the infant-lessons learned. J Urol 2006;176:2237–9 [discussion: 2239–40].

28. Lee RS, Retik AB, Borer JG, et al. Pediatric robot assisted laparoscopic dismembered pyeloplasty: comparison with a cohort of open surgery. J Urol 2006;175:683–7 [discussion: 687].

29. Yee DS, Shanberg AM, Duel BP, et al. Initial comparison of robotic-assisted laparoscopic versus open pyeloplasty in children. Urology 2006;67:599–602.

30. Olsen LH, Rawashdeh YF, Jorgensen TM. Pediatric robot assisted retroperitoneoscopic pyeloplasty: a 5-year experience. J Urol 2007;178:2137–41 [discussion: 2141].

31. Franco I, Dyer LL, Zelkovic P. Laparoscopic pyeloplasty in the pediatric patient: hand sewn anastomosis versus robotic assisted anastomosis–is there a difference? J Urol 2007;178:1483–6.

32. Freilich DA, Nguyen HT, Borer J, et al. Concurrent management of bilateral ureteropelvic junction obstruction in children using robotic-assisted laparoscopic surgery. Int Braz J Urol 2008;34:198–204 [discussion: 204–5].

33. Chan KW, Lee KH, Tam YH, et al. Early experience of robotic-assisted reconstructive operations in pediatric urology. J Laparoendosc Adv Surg Tech A 2010; 20:379–82.

34. Steinberg PL, Merguerian PA, Bihrle W 3rd, et al. The cost of learning robotic-assisted prostatectomy. Urology 2008;72:1068–72.

35. Tasian GE, Wiebe DJ, Casale P. Learning curve of robotic assisted pyeloplasty for pediatric urology fellows. J Urol 2013;190:1622–6.

36. Kilic GS, Walsh TM, Borahay M, et al. Effect of residents' previous laparoscopic surgery experience on initial robotic suturing experience. ISRN Obstet Gynecol 2012;2012:569456.

37. O'Brien ST, Shukla AR. Transition from open to robotic-assisted pediatric pyeloplasty: a feasibility and outcome study. J Pediatr Urol 2012;8:276–81.

The Robotic-assisted Ureteral Reimplantation
The Evolution to a New Standard

Dana A. Weiss, MD*, Aseem R. Shukla, MD

KEYWORDS

- Robotic-assisted laparoscopic ureteral reimplantation • Extravesical • Intravesical

KEY POINTS

- Robotic-assisted laparoscopic ureteral reimplantation is a safe and efficacious alternative to open ureteral reimplantation.
- Careful attention to dissection of the distal ureter and creation of the detrusor tunnel can minimize postoperative urinary retention and bladder irritation.
- Robotic ureteral reimplantation can be used not only for vesicoureteral reflux but also for treatment of distal ureteral obstruction.

INTRODUCTION: NATURE OF THE PROBLEM

Vesicoureteral reflux, the retrograde flow of urine from the bladder into the ureters and the renal collecting system, is a commonly encountered anomaly in the pediatric urology practice. Diagnosis is generally rendered with a voiding cystourethrogram (VCUG) as a result of an evaluation for prenatal dilation of the urinary tract, or a febrile urinary tract infection (UTI). The incidence of vesicoureteral reflux has been shown to be 30% to 50% in children presenting with at least 1 UTI, and about 15% to 41% in children undergoing a workup for antenatally detected hydronephrosis.[1,2] Although not all cases of vesicoureteral reflux need to be repaired, in cases of recurrent infection or persistent high-grade reflux, surgical correction is a potential intervention to prevent pyelonephritis and renal scarring.[3,4]

Options for repair of vesicoureteral reflux include the following:

- Endoscopic injection (Deflux or other bulking agents; Salix Pharmaceuticals, Raleigh, NC, USA)
- Open intravesical reimplantation
- Open extravesical reimplantation
- Minimally invasive (laparoscopic or robotic-assisted) intravesical reimplantation
- Minimally invasive (laparoscopic or robotic-assisted) extravesical reimplantation

Open intravesical ureteral reimplantation is widely considered the "gold-standard" approach for the correction of vesicoureteral reflux because of historical success rates that range from 95% to 99%.[5,6] The limitation to these statistics, however, is that some studies comprise cohorts without a postoperative VCUG and others had variations in patient selection. Indeed, some more recent studies imply a lower success rate of around 93%, when a VCUG was rigorously completed 3 months postoperatively.[7] Despite the popularity and widespread reliance on the intraoperative open reimplantation, commonly encountered postoperative symptoms inherent to a procedure relying on an open cystotomy—hematuria, bladder spasms, and irritative voiding symptoms—have encouraged surgeons to explore alternatives.[3,8] One such alternative has always been the open extravesical ureteral reimplantation. However, this too has drawback of requiring an open Pfannenstiel incision and carries the risk of postoperative

Division of Urology, The Children's Hospital of Philadelphia, Wood Building, 3rd Floor, 34th and Civic Center Boulevard, Philadelphia, PA 19104, USA
* Corresponding author.
E-mail address: weissd1@email.chop.edu

Urol Clin N Am 42 (2015) 99–109
http://dx.doi.org/10.1016/j.ucl.2014.09.010

urologic.theclinics.com

urinary retention, thought to be due to a neuropraxia from dissection around the bladder.[9,10] Indeed, the urge to avoid this neuropraxia has led most urologists to prefer the open extravesical approach only in unilateral procedures rather than in bilateral procedures.

Urology, as a specialty, has traditionally positioned itself at the intersection of technology and surgery and has been an early adaptor of minimally invasive surgery, ever since the first lap nephrectomy in 1991. Not long after, the first pediatric laparoscopic extravesical reimplantation was described in 1994.[8,11] Following this, urologists further innovated with the laparoscopic intravesical Cohen cross-trigonal reimplant.[12] However, because of a steep learning curve and considerable physical strain on the surgeon—exacerbated in smaller children—the pure laparoscopic approach was not broadly accepted. Although variations in surgical technique have been reported, overall, results were not as consistent as the open technique and procedures were complicated by urinary fistulae and bladder leaks.[3,12–17]

The advent of the da Vinci Surgical System (Intuitive Surgical, Mountain View, CA, USA) revolutionized minimally invasive surgery. The da Vinci system, using a master-slave platform that is under the control of the surgeon, carries well-known advantages of 3-dimensional visualization (now in high definition), articulating instruments and dampening of tremor. The robotic-assisted laparoscopic (RAL) surgery concept has facilitated the use of minimally invasive approaches in both adults and children and is in widespread use for procedures ranging from the radical prostatectomy to reconstructive urology.[18] Peters and Woo[14] described the robotic-assisted transvesicoscopic approach, where only 1 patient of 6 initial patients had a complication of a urine leak. The inherent challenges of obtaining and maintaining pneumovesicum, and the challenges of limited articulation of robotic instrumentation in the bladder, limited popularity of the intravesical technique. However one of the earliest large series of RAL extravesical ureteral reimplantations in 2008 reported success equivalent to those generally expected by the open technique.[12] As demonstrated herein, the use of the RAL surgery has made the repair of vesicoureteral reflux a viable approach in comparison with antibiotic prophylaxis, even as the potential adverse events are mitigated by improved magnification and focused dissection.[9,14,19]

INDICATIONS/CONTRAINDICATIONS

For vesicoureteral reflux (VUR), indications for treatment include recurrent pyelonephritis/febrile UTIs, worsening hydronephrosis/parenchymal thinning, worsening function on renal scan, and desire by parents to come off of prophylactic antibiotics. However, the technique of RAL ureteral reimplantation (RALUR) is applicable for the correction of VUR and the same approach may be used for other interventions as well. Indications for RALUR also include management of obstructed megaureters and distal ureteral strictures resulting in loss of function, pain, UTI, and sepsis. For these, the repair of the obstructed distal ureter requires a dismembered reimplantation to excise the narrowed ureterovesical junction followed by reanastomosis of the ureter to the bladder and creation of a nonrefluxing tunnel.[20] There are very few definite contraindications to RALUR—primarily lung or heart anomalies that preclude insufflation. Even a history of previous abdominal surgery is only a relative contraindication to laparoscopy—a rare occurrence when significant adhesions preclude safe access to the abdominal cavity.

TECHNIQUE/PROCEDURE
Preparation

Preoperative assessment is the same regardless of whether the surgical approach will be vesicoscopic or extravesical. Appropriate imaging including ultrasound, VCUG, and dimercaptosuccinic acid (optional) should be reviewed before surgery. Routine preoperative laboratory tests are not required, but a urinalysis or urine culture is recommended if the patient has been symptomatic recently. Patient size does not limit the use of the robotic approach; however, for the intravesical approach, it is advisable that the patient be more than 4 years of age with a bladder capacity of at least 200 mL.[21]

Patient Positioning

The patient is placed supine in the low lithotomy position on Allen stirrups, which allow for preoperative cystourethroscopy in the same setting, if required. For smaller patients, the patient can remain supine with the legs on the table as well. The patient is secured to the bed with taping across the chest, with care to assure that all pressure points are well padded. In addition, it is recommended to be careful here to ensure that the head of the patient is turned to the side to avoid the robotic arms hitting the endotracheal tube. A sterile preparation of the abdomen from xyphoid down through perineum is performed, and the patient is draped, so that there is access to the urethra for cystourethroscopy or catheter placement during the procedure. The authors find a sketch over the drape overlying the child's head makes everyone cognizant of where the face and tube are during the procedure.

Approach

For all ureteral reimplantations where dismemberment of the ureterovesical junction is foreseen, as in cases of obstructed megaureter or ureteral stenosis, start by performing cystoscopy with ureteral stent placement. Some surgeons prefer to place ureteral stents temporarily during extravesical ureteral reimplantation as well, so this is done at the beginning of the procedure. Ureteral stent placement is not standard practice for most cases.

Intravesical Robotic-assisted Ureteral Reimplant: Technique

The patient is placed into a steep Trendelenberg position at the start of the procedure. The bladder is filled with saline and the ports are placed under constant direct cystoscopic vision. Before port placement, 2 sutures are passed transabdominally through the rectus fascia and into the bladder under cystoscopic guidance. These sutures are used to keep the bladder tented to the abdominal wall during the surgery and then are used to close the bladder at the end of the operation. Initially, a transverse midline incision below the umbilicus is made for the camera port (8.5 mm). This port is positioned in the dome of the bladder. The 2 robotic working arms are placed at the edge of the rectus on each side, just below the level of the camera port. Once all ports are placed, the saline is emptied from the bladder and the bladder is filled with CO_2.

Ureteral stents are placed into the bladder through one of the robotic ports and then advanced into the ureter. Ureteral stents are then sutured to the ureteral orifice with a monofilament suture. The stent and suture are then used as a handle for manipulating the ureter during mobilization. Just as in an open repair, the ureter is mobilized from the level of the orifice through the intramural region into the retroperitoneum.[21] A feeding tube placed transurethrally and connected to suction can be used intermittently as a suctioning device and then clamped when not in use.[15,22]

Once the ureter is mobilized, the opening in the detrusor is closed to prevent loss of the pneumovesical pressure. A submucosal tunnel is then created by sharp dissection with cold scissors or it can be made by tunneling a ureteral dilator. The ureteral stent is then passed through the tunnel first, and the ureter is pulled along in suit.

Finally, the ureteral cuff is sutured to the bladder mucosa in an interrupted fashion. Ureteral stents can be left depending on the surgeon's preference.

Postoperative recovery is the same as with most minimally invasive surgery in pediatric urology. A VCUG is performed on the day after surgery to rule out a bladder leak, and if negative, the Foley catheter can be removed.[21]

Extravesical Robotic-assisted Ureteral Reimplant: Technique

After the patient has been prepared and draped in the aforementioned manner, a Foley catheter is placed in sterile fashion on the field and a urine culture is obtained. Intraperitoneal access is obtained at the umbilicus (curvilinear incision at the inferior umbilicus or vertical incision through the umbilicus.) Here, via the Veress or Hassan technique, the 8.5-mm robotic port is placed. Next, the table is placed into the steep Trendelenberg position to allow all peritoneal contents to slide cranially. Two robotic 5-mm ports are positioned below the level of the umbilicus in the midclavicular line. If performing a unilateral reimplant, then the ports can be skewed so that the ipsilateral port is placed more cephalad than the contralateral side to improve the working distance on that side and to maximize triangulation toward the region of interest. The authors generally use a hook on the right and a Maryland grasper on the left; however, some surgeons prefer 8-mm ports and thus can use the hot scissors on the right instead.

The dissection begins by opening the peritoneum; in female patients, dissection begins distal to the round ligament to visualize the ureter and then proceeds proximally from there (**Fig. 1**). In male patients, the ureter is first visualized and this is traced distally until the vas deferens is identified. The peritoneum is opened distal to the vas with careful attention to sweep the vas away from the surgical field to avoid injury. The ureter is dissected distally to the level of the ureterovesical junction, and proximally until there is good freedom of movement with minimal tension when lifted toward the bladder.

The authors use a transabdominal wall hitch stitch (0 polydiaxanone (PDS II, Ethicon) on CT 1 needle) placed into the bladder to provide superior tension for better visibility and handling of the bladder for the dissection and repair (**Fig. 2**). The bladder is filled via the urethral catheter with 30 to 50 cc saline. With hook cautery, the detrusor is incised vertically, making sure not to enter the mucosa. The incision is extended all the way

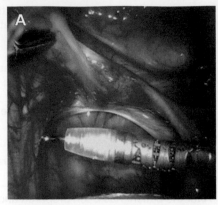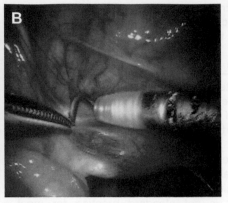

Fig. 1. (A) Identification of ureter in female. (B) Opening peritoneum distal to broad ligament.

down to the ureter anteriorly, but the authors do not dissect circumferentially around the ureter. The tunnel is made at a length of 4 or 5:1 of the diameter of the ureter. During the dissection, a "blue dome" of mucosa protrudes, and this enables visualization of each individual detrusor fiber, because it is important to cut all detrusor fibers of bladder thoroughly. Finally, the authors develop flaps of detrusor on either side that will be used to close over the ureter (Fig. 3).

Once the ureter and bladder are ready, the detrusorrhaphy is begun. Using 5-0 poliglecaprone (Monocryl, Ethicon, Blue Ash, OH, USA) suture (this is the authors' preference, because it has less memory than polydiaxonone, PDS II, Ethicon), the edges of the detrusor are approximated from the level of the ureteropelvic junction superiorly. After taking a stitch of the detrusor flap on one side, these sutures are passed underneath the ureter to the contralateral detrusor flap to ensure advancement of the ureter within the detrusor trough. To complete the stitch, the needle is again passed back under the ureter to the original side and tied there (Fig. 4). For the first 2 stitches, a very small bite of adventitia of the ureter is taken, to prevent the ureter from slipping out of the tunnel.

Alternatively, some surgeons prefer to affix the ureter to the distal end of the detrusor trough with the first suture pass and then close the detrusor over the top of the ureter. The authors prefer the gradual closure from bottom to top to assess tension at every step. Caution here is required as taking too much of a bite on the ureteral adventitia can cause obstruction, and taking the ureter up too high in the tunnel can kink the ureter and cause obstruction as well. As a last step, the hitch stitch is released and the ureter and bladder position are assessed.

Finall robotic ports are removed and the fascia and skin of all ports are closed. The authors prefer to use local anesthetic injection in individual port sites rather than a preoperative intrathecal opiate injection because, in the authors' experience, the local anesthetic has similar efficacy while avoiding potential complications of a central block.

Complications and Management

Complications of robotic ureteral reimplant include the following:

- Bleeding: With careful ureteral dissection, bleeding is very rare. Most often point

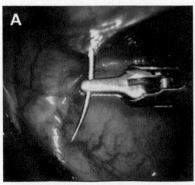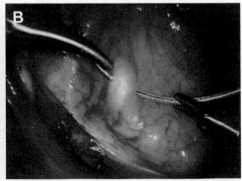

Fig. 2. (A) Needle of hitch stitch being passed through anterior abdominal wall. (B) Placing hitch stitch through bladder.

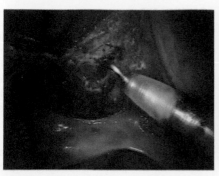
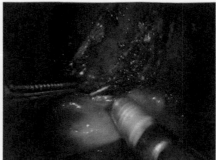

Fig. 3. Incision of depressor, with visualization of "blue dome" (right).

coagulation and pressure can control bleeding encountered during the surgery.

- Bowel injury: This can occur during intraperitoneal access, as in any laparoscopic case. The key to this is early identification, because most injuries are small and can be managed by primary closure or oversewing a segment. The other area of risk is of inadvertent thermal injury by the camera or by a robotic arm during coagulation. Unfortunately, most of these have a delayed presentation of 2 to 3 days, manifested by abdominal pain, fever, and leukocytosis. Port-site pain is the classic indicator of an intraperitoneal injury and mandates a full evaluation. A high index of suspicion for this is necessary for diagnosis.
- Ileus: This is not uncommon postoperatively and is usually mild in nature with self-resolution within 1 to 2 days. Focus on decreasing narcotic use and early ambulation may help to prevent this.
- Port-site hernia: This usually has a delayed presentation after 2 to 3 weeks. It may present as an asymptomatic bulge or pain at a port site (**Fig. 5**). The diagnosis can be confirmed with ultrasound, and management involves surgical reduction and closure of the fascia.

This repair may be performed laparoscopically with simple reduction of the omental tissue that is the typical herniated content. The fascia of all 3 port sites should be closed at the time of surgery, but this does not prevent hernia in all cases.

- Ureteral obstruction: This is most often due to transient edema and can be managed expectantly if the patient is still making urine. In the setting of a solitary kidney, a ureteral stent should be left at the time of surgery. If obstruction does not improve or the patient becomes anuric, urgent placement of a ureteral stent is required.
- Ureteral injury: This can be due to aggressive dissection and devascularization of the ureter or due to an inadvertent incision in the ureter. A ureteral injury may be noticed intraoperatively or may have a delayed presentation. Because postoperative drains are not used, abdominal distention and pain, and ileus may be signs of injury. Laboratory values of increased serum creatinine (because of urine absorption) and renal bladder ultrasound findings of free intra-abdominal fluid with or without hydronephrosis may indicate the need for further investigation.

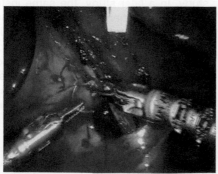
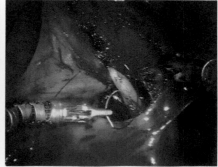

Fig. 4. Detrussor closure with passage of suture needle underneath ureter (right).

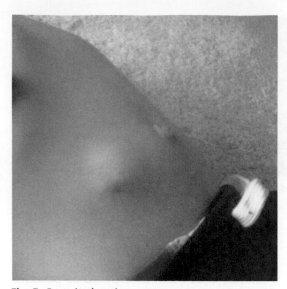

Fig. 5. Port site hernia.

- Urinary retention: This is the most common complication after ureteral reimplantation. To avoid this, surgeons may consider leaving a suprapubic tube at the time of surgery in patients with known dysfunctional voiding. Alternatively, a Foley catheter can be kept for several days in these children to avoid replacement. Once the Foley catheter is removed, the child should be encouraged to timed void every 2 to 3 hours to promote bladder emptying.

Postoperative Care

Although this surgery can be performed on an outpatient basis, most children are kept in the hospital for one night with a Foley catheter in place. Diet is begun immediately and advanced as tolerated, but the child is kept on intravenous fluids until they are able to tolerate oral intake sufficiently. The Foley catheter is removed the next morning, and the patient can be discharged once she is able to urinate with a residual that is less than 1/2 of the total volume voided.

Follow-Up

The patient returns to clinic in 1 month with an ultrasound. If no abnormalities are detected, prophylactic antibiotics are then discontinued at that point. Because a pilot study by surgeons at the authors' institution revealed a sufficiently high resolution rate by the RALUR technique, the authors do not routinely perform a postoperative VCUG study unless the child develops another recurrent febrile UTI.[23]

OUTCOMES

Table 1 displays results from a wide range of studies that have been performed to evaluate the safety and efficacy of the RALUR. The studies clearly reveal that current practice trends easily favor RALUR over pure laparoscopy, likely due to the former's benefits in increased range of motion, ease of suturing, and improved ergonomics rendering less strain on the surgeon.

Kutikov and colleagues[15] reported on an experience of 27 patients undergoing the laparoscopic transvesical ureteral reimplantation for vesicoureteral reflux (as well as an additional 5 for primary obstructed megaureter). Four of the 27 reflux operations had complications including postoperative ureteral leak and development of a ureteral stricture. Three of the 4 patients who had complications had small bladders, which highlighted a key factor of bladder size that affected outcomes.

In a direct comparison between open and pure laparoscopic vesicoscopic ureteral reimplants, Canon and colleagues[24] retrospectively reviewed 52 patients who underwent vesicoscopic, and 40 who underwent open ureteral reimplantations. There were 3 complications in the vesicoscopic group compared with 0 in the open, and resolution of VUR was only in 91% versus 97%. However, this was still an early experience, and later, Valla and colleagues[25] reported a 95% success rate in 72 vesicoscopic reimplants.

With the advent of robotics to enable more complex laparoscopic reconstructive procedures, the technology has been increasingly implemented in the pediatric population as well. In 2008, Casale and colleagues[9] reported their experience of bilateral extravesical RALUR. In this series of 41 patients, there were 8 patients with grade 3 VUR, 5 patients with grade 4, and 5 patients with grade 5 VUR. No patient experienced postoperative urinary retention, and there was resolution in 40 of 41 (97.6%) as confirmed by postoperative VCUG study. In a later study, the same institution presented 150 patients followed prospectively and treated with bilateral extravesical RALUR for grade 3 or higher VUR. Here, they identified no complications and reported a 99.3% VUR resolution rate based on postoperative VCUG studies.[26] The authors think that the ×10 magnification and 3D visualization of the robotic console aids in identifying nerve bundles that minimize the risk of postoperative urinary retention.

In 2011, Smith and colleagues[13] presented a comparative study of 25 RALUR matched with 25 open cross-trigonal ureteral reimplantations.

For outcomes, a VCUG was performed for all robotic reimplants, while the lack of a febrile UTI was considered success for the open group. In this head-to-head comparison, RALUR was found to be safe and efficacious. They found that the open group had statistically significantly lower operative time, but the RALUR group had shorter length of stay and diminished postoperative analgesic use. When comparing only those who had postoperative VCUG in each group, the robotic group had a 96% resolution rate, whereas the open group resolved in 100% of cases. Of note, 3 of the 8 children in the bilateral extravesical RALUR group did experience transient postoperative retention.

Marchini and colleagues[7] directly compared RALUR using the vesicoscopic or extravesical approach, as well as pure laparoscopic extravesical reimplantations. By setting up a retrospective 4-way matched comparison between both open and laparoscopic intravesical and extravesical approaches, the group found that operative time was significantly lower for both open intravesical and extravesical procedures, while hospital stay was lower in the robotic intravesical group compared with the open intravesical group. Both RALUR groups with extravesical approaches had the same length of stay. There was a higher incidence of bladder spasms in the open intravesical group compared with any other group, while each of the RALUR groups—intravesical and extravesical—did see cases of urinary retention (1 intravesical and 2 extravesical) not seen in the open groups. Four patients in the robotic intravesical group had bladder leaks, and 2 undergoing robotic extravesical reimplants had ureteral leaks. At 3-month follow-up with VCUG, 3 in the robotic intravesical reimplant group and 4 in the open (3 in the intravesical and 1 in the extravesical) group had VUR.

In a small single-surgeon experience with RALUR, Chalmers and colleagues[27] presented results for 23 ureters with a 90.9% success rate, underscoring the importance of a sufficiently long tunnel. Calculating tunnel length during the transition from open to minimally invasive surgery is technically challenging because of the obviously different optical dimensions and requires careful measurement using instruments with known lengths as a reference, or a measuring tape that can be inserted during the procedure.

In a recent report, Akhavan and colleagues[28] presented a retrospective experience of 78 ureters in 50 patients over 7 years that underwent RALUR using the extravesical approach. Most of these repairs were done for grade 3 VUR,

and some required bilateral procedures. All patients not only underwent US postoperatively but also underwent postoperative radionuclide cystograms to assess resolution of VUR. This cohort had a 92.3% success rate (defined as no residual VUR). A total of 10% of patients did experience a postoperative UTI, but none of these were found to have residual VUR. All patients developing a postoperative UTI were girls with a history of detrusor external sphincter dyssynergia. A total of 2% of the entire group and 4% of the bilateral RALUR group did experience urinary retention even for up to 3 weeks. These patients had been identified preoperatively as having voiding dysfunction, and suprapubic tubes were placed preemptively at the time of surgery. Up to 10% of patients had complications including edema causing transient ureteral obstruction, ileus, perinephric fluid collection, and ureteral injury. All obstructions and leaks were treated with ureteral stent placement.

Finally, Schomburg and colleagues[23] presented an experience of a single surgeon performing open extravesical reimplantations compared with extravesical RALUR. In this matched comparison of 20 patients in each group, they found that the procedure did take longer in the robotic cohort for both unilateral and bilateral procedures (165 min vs 109 min for the unilateral, and 227 min vs 134.5 min for bilateral, $P<.001$), but there was no difference in duration of urethral catheterization, length of stay, postoperative retention, or persistent VUR. The robotic group did use fewer morphine equivalents for postoperative pain control. There was no difference in complication rates in each group.

CURRENT CONTROVERSIES/FUTURE CONSIDERATIONS

Minimally invasive surgical techniques carry the necessary burden of proving that the benefits of improved cosmesis and decreased analgesia are not predicated on compromised safety or efficacy. It may be rightfully argued that the RALUR has been proven as feasible, safe, and efficacious while delivering the well-known benefit of minimally invasive surgery. The long-term durability and safety of the repair, which is comparable to open repairs in the near term, await substantiation. Last, surgeons must continue to ensure that the technological leapfrogging does not begin to change the indications for surgery. The technology must be used as a tool—as a means to an end rather than use the technology as a means in and of itself.

Table 1
Results from studies evaluating the safety and efficacy of the robot-assisted laparoscopic ureteral reimplantation

Study	Technique	Patients (n)/ Ureters (n)	Mean/Median Age (Range), y	Mean/Median Operative Time, h	Mean/Median LOS (Range), d	Complications	Success (%)
Peters and Woo,[14] 2005	RALUR/IV	6/12	5/15	NA	2-4	1(urine leak)	83.3
Kutikov et al,[15] 2006	LUR/IV	27 (54)[a]	5 (1.2–11)	2.8	45.7 (22–92)	3 (leak = 2, stricture = 1) (tapered ureter)	92.6
Canon et al,[24] 2007	LUR/IV OR/IV	52 LUR/40 OR	5.7/4.0	LUR/IV 3.3 OR/IV 1.5	LUR/IV 2.1 OR/IV 2.0	3 (LUR): (urinary leak = 1, stones = 1, bilateral ureteral obstruction = 1)	91 (LUR)/97 (OR)
Valla et al,[25] 2009	LUR/IV	72	4.2 (0.5–14)	1.37 uni/2.17 bil	2.8	6 (2, abdominal wall hematoma, 4, converted to open)[b]	95%
Marchini et al,[7] 2011	RALUR/IV and EV OR/IV and EV	RALUR 19 intra 20 extra Open 22 intra 17 extra	RALUR intra, 9.9 RALUR extra, 8.6 Open intra, 8.8 Open extra,6.0	RALUR intra, 3.88 RALUR extra, 3.89 Open intra, 2.46 Open extra, 2.0	RALUR/IV 1.8 RALUR/EV 1.7 OR/IV 2.9 OR/EV 1.7	RI, 5 (retention =1, leak, 4), RE, 4 (retention = 2, ureteral leak = 2), OI, 0, OE, 0[c]	RALUR/IV 92.2 RALUR/EV 100 OR/IV 93.2 OR/EV 94.2
Emir et al,[29] 2012	LUR/IV	11 (17)	6.9 (2–15)	3.61/5.1	3.8 (3–5)	0	94

Casale et al,[9] 2008	RALUR/EV	41 (82)	3.2 (1.3–6.8)	2.33	26.1	0	97.6
Smith et al,[13] 2011	RALUR/EV OR/IV	RALUR/EV 25 (33) OR/IV 25 (46)	5.8/4.2	3.08/2.75	33/51	4 (3, urinary retention, in bilateral RALUR; 1, bladder leak in OR)	RALUR/EV 97 OR/IV 100
Kasturi et al,[26] 2012	RALUR/EV	150 (300)	3.55 (2.25–9.25)	1.8	22.1 (18–34)	0	99.3
Chalmers et al,[27] 2012	RALUR/EV	17 (23)	6.23 ± 3.4	2.12/2.95	1.3	0	90.9
Bayne et al,[30] 2012	LUR/EV	98 (144)	6 (0.9–20.3)	NA	1.35	4 (retention = 3, obstruction = 1)	95.2
Schomburg et al,[23] 2014	RALUR/EV OR/EV	20 RALUR 20 OR	6.2, RALUR/EV 4.3 OR/EV	RALUR uni, 2.75 RALUR bil, 3.78 Open uni, 1.82 Open bil, 2.23	RALUR/EV 1.05 OR/EV 1.4	RALUR, 2, OR, 7	RALUR/EV 100[d] OR/EV 95
Akhavan et al,[28] 2014	RALUR/EV	50 (78)	6.2 (1.9–18.0)	NA	2.0 (1–6)	6 (ileus = 2, ureteral obstruction = 2, ureteral injury = 1, perinephric fluid = 1)	92.3

Abbreviations: EV, extravesical; IV, intravesical; LUR, laparoscopic ureteral reimplant; OR, open ureteral reimplant.

[a] Excludes surgeries in series performed for primary obstructed megaureter.
[b] Excluded spontaneously resolving scrotal emphysema, pneumoperitoneum intraoperatively.
[c] Excluded pain greater than 2, bladder spasms, and hematuria from complication list.
[d] Not all RALUR had postoperative VCUG.

SUMMARY

- RALUR is a safe and efficacious alternative to open ureteral reimplantation.
- Careful attention to dissection of the distal ureter and creation of the detrusor tunnel can minimize postoperative urinary retention and bladder irritation.
- Robotic ureteral reimplantation can be used not only for vesicoureteral reflux but also for treatment of distal ureteral obstruction.

REFERENCES

1. van Eerde AM, Meutgeert MH, de Jong TP, et al. Vesico-ureteral reflux in children with prenatally detected hydronephrosis: a systematic review. Ultrasound Obstet Gynecol 2007;29:463–9.
2. Moorthy I, Joshi N, Cook JV, et al. Antenatal hydronephrosis: negative predictive value of normal postnatal ultrasound–a 5-year study. Clin Radiol 2003; 58:964–70.
3. Trevisani LF, Nguyen HT. Current controversies in pediatric urologic robotic surgery. Curr Opin Urol 2013;23:72–7.
4. Elder JS. Guidelines for consideration for surgical repair of vesicoureteral reflux. Curr Opin Urol 2000; 10:579–85.
5. Skoog SJ, Peters CA, Arant BS Jr, et al. Pediatric vesicoureteral reflux guidelines panel summary report: clinical practice guidelines for screening siblings of children with vesicoureteral reflux and neonates/infants with prenatal hydronephrosis. J Urol 2010;184:1145–51.
6. McCool AC, Joseph DB. Postoperative hospitalization of children undergoing cross-trigonal ureteroneocystostomy. J Urol 1995;154:794–6.
7. Marchini GS, Hong YK, Minnillo BJ, et al. Robotic assisted laparoscopic ureteral reimplantation in children: case matched comparative study with open surgical approach. J Urol 2011;185: 1870–5.
8. Ehrlich RM, Gershman A, Fuchs G. Laparoscopic vesicoureteroplasty in children: initial case reports. Urology 1994;43:255–61.
9. Casale P, Patel RP, Kolon TF. Nerve sparing robotic extravesical ureteral reimplantation. J Urol 2008; 179:1987–9 [discussion: 90].
10. Dangle PP, Razmaria AA, Towle VL, et al. Is pelvic plexus nerve documentation feasible during robotic assisted laparoscopic ureteral reimplantation with extravesical approach? J Pediatr Urol 2013; 9:442–7.
11. Janetschek G, Radmayr C, Bartsch G. Laparoscopic ureteral anti-reflux plasty reimplantation. First clinical experience. Ann Urol (Paris) 1995;29: 101–5.

12. Gill IS, Ponsky LE, Desai M, et al. Laparoscopic cross-trigonal Cohen ureteroneocystostomy: novel technique. J Urol 2001;166:1811–4.
13. Smith RP, Oliver JL, Peters CA. Pediatric robotic extravesical ureteral reimplantation: comparison with open surgery. J Urol 2011;185:1876–81.
14. Peters CA, Woo R. Intravesical robotically assisted bilateral ureteral reimplantation. J Endourol 2005; 19:618–21 [discussion: 21–2].
15. Kutikov A, Guzzo TJ, Canter DJ, et al. Initial experience with laparoscopic transvesical ureteral reimplantation at the Children's Hospital of Philadelphia. J Urol 2006;176:2222–5 [discussion: 5–6].
16. Cartwright PC, Snow BW, Mansfield JC, et al. Percutaneous endoscopic trigonoplasty: a minimally invasive approach to correct vesicoureteral reflux. J Urol 1996;156:661–4.
17. Tsuji Y, Okamura K, Nishimura T, et al. A new endoscopic ureteral reimplantation for primary vesicoureteral reflux (endoscopic trigonoplasty II). J Urol 2003;169:1020–2.
18. Phillips EA, Wang DS. Current status of robot-assisted laparoscopic ureteral reimplantation and reconstruction. Curr Urol Rep 2012;13:190–4.
19. Mathews R, Carpenter M, Chesney R, et al. Controversies in the management of vesicoureteral reflux: the rationale for the RIVUR study. J Pediatr Urol 2009;5:336–41.
20. Faasse MA, Lindgren BW, Gong EM. Robot-assisted laparoscopic ureteral reimplantation with excisional tailoring for refluxing megaureter. J Pediatr Urol 2014. [Epub ahead of print].
21. Minnillo BJ, Marchini GS, Nguyen HT. Robotic-assisted intravesical ureteral reimplantation. In: Gundeti MS, editor. Pediatric robotic and reconstructive urology: a comprehensive guide. Hoboken (NJ): Wiley-Blackwell; 2012. p. 151–9.
22. Yeung CK, Sihoe JD, Borzi PA. Endoscopic cross-trigonal ureteral reimplantation under carbon dioxide bladder insufflation: a novel technique. J Endourol 2005;19:295–9.
23. Schomburg JL, Haberman K, Willihnganz-Lawson KH, et al. Robot-assisted laparoscopic ureteral reimplantation: a single surgeon comparison to open surgery. J Pediatr Urol 2014. [Epub ahead of print].
24. Canon SJ, Jayanthi VR, Patel AS. Vesicoscopic cross-trigonal ureteral reimplantation: a minimally invasive option for repair of vesicoureteral reflux. J Urol 2007;178:269–73 [discussion: 73].
25. Valla JS, Steyaert H, Griffin SJ, et al. Transvesicoscopic Cohen ureteric reimplantation for vesicoureteral reflux in children: a single-centre 5-year experience. J Pediatr Urol 2009;5:466–71.
26. Kasturi S, Sehgal SS, Christman MS, et al. Prospective long-term analysis of nerve-sparing extravesical robotic-assisted laparoscopic ureteral reimplantation. Urology 2012;79:680–3.

27. Chalmers D, Herbst K, Kim C. Robotic-assisted laparoscopic extravesical ureteral reimplantation: an initial experience. J Pediatr Urol 2012;8: 268–71.

28. Akhavan A, Avery D, Lendvay TS. Robot-assisted extravesical ureteral reimplantation: outcomes and conclusions from 78 ureters. J Pediatr Urol 2014. [Epub ahead of print].

29. Emir H, Mammadov E, Elicevik M, et al. Transvesicoscopic cross-trigonal ureteroneocystostomy in children: a single-center experience. J Pediatr Urol 2012;8:83–6.

30. Bayne AP, Shoss JM, Starke NR, et al. Single-center experience with pediatric laparoscopic extravesical reimplantation: safe and effective in simple and complex anatomy. J Laparoendosc Adv Surg Tech A 2012;22:102–6.

Robotic-Assisted Bladder Neck Repair
Feasibility and Outcomes

Patricio C. Gargollo, MD

KEYWORDS

- Robotic surgery • Urinary incontinence • Bladder neck reconstruction • Neurogenic bladder
- Appendicovesicostomy

KEY POINTS

- Complex robotic reconstruction follows the same steps and principles as those used during open surgery.
- Robotic bladder neck reconstruction is safe and feasible.
- Surgeons should expect longer operative times during robotic bladder neck reconstruction when compared with open.
- Patients with multiple ventriculo-peritoneal (VP) shunt revisions at the abdominal level have a statistically higher rate of intra-abdominal adhesions and higher conversion rates.

Minimally invasive techniques are rapidly being developed and integrated into urologic surgery. Over the past 5 years, the urologic literature is abound with novel techniques and adaptations to conventional laparoscopy, including but not limited to laparoendoscopic single-site surgery, natural orifice transluminal endoscopic surgery, and robot-assisted laparoscopic surgery (RALS). Pediatric urology is no exception to this trend, and the benefits of minimally invasive surgery may be accentuated in children given the relatively more confined working spaces and also a heightened awareness of cosmesis for the pediatric population. Increasingly, complex pediatric urologic procedures are being performed with robot assistance. The feasibility of nephrectomy, pyeloplasty, ureteral reimplantation, and bladder surgery has been clearly established. A few case reports and a small series have been published describing robot-assisted Mitrofanoff appendicovesicostomy (APV) with or without augmentation ileocystoplasty or creation of an anterograde continent enema colon tube.[1–3]

SURGICAL INTERVENTION FOR URINARY INCONTINENCE

Urinary incontinence secondary to an incompetent urethral sphincter mechanism is an entity commonly encountered in pediatric urology with multiple etiologies. Regardless of the primary cause (exstrophy/epispadias, cloacal anomalies, or neurogenic bladder secondary to spinal cord injury or dysraphisms) urine leakage in the absence of a detrusor contraction is the definition of an incompetent urinary sphincter mechanism.[4] It is in this patient population that a bladder outlet procedure, with possible concomitant procedures depending on the patient, is indicated to achieve urinary continence. Whether or not a concomitant bladder augmentation procedure should be performed is a highly contested topic and beyond the scope of this article, and thus will not be covered here.

The essential mechanism behind all surgical procedures for urinary incontinence secondary to an incompetent sphincter is to somehow tighten the bladder outlet. This can be accomplished

Urology Robotic and Minimally Invasive Surgery Program, Division of Pediatric Urology, Department of Surgery, Baylor College of Medicine, Center for Complex Urogenital Reconstruction, Texas Children's Hospital, 6701 Fannin Street, 6th Floor, Houston, TX 77030, USA
E-mail address: pcgargol@texaschildrens.org

Urol Clin N Am 42 (2015) 111–120
http://dx.doi.org/10.1016/j.ucl.2014.09.013
0094-0143/15/$ – see front matter © 2015 Elsevier Inc. All rights reserved.

through placement of a sling or artificial urinary sphincter or through a bladder neck reconstruction (BNR). In some cases, a bladder neck closure also can be performed. At our institution, management of neurogenic bladder with persistent urinary incontinence, despite clean intermittent catheterization (CIC) and anticholinergic therapy, includes creation of a Mitrofanoff APV (or Monti channel when the appendix is inadequate) and Leadbetter/Mitchell (LM) BNR along with a bladder neck sling (BNS).[5] Currently our center is one of a few performing these reconstructions using RALS. Because of this there is a paucity of data on robotic outcomes, we will thus first present some data from open series.

OUTCOMES FROM OPEN SERIES
Bladder Neck Repairs

There are various bladder neck reconstructive procedures that are available to increase the resistance at the bladder outlet. Perhaps the most common are the Young-Dees Leadbetter (YDL), the Pippi-Salle, the Kropp repair, and the modified LM repair.[6] Various studies have looked at outcomes with these different techniques, but unfortunately all of the published literature suffers from multiple limitations, including retrospective studies with significant confounders, nonstandardized protocols, and multiple definitions of what constitutes urinary continence. Most articles also combine patients with different primary diagnoses and some do not differentiate between BNR with and without augmentation cystoplasty. For example, in a retrospective study of 49 continence procedures in patients with multiple etiologies for their incontinence, Cole and colleagues[7] showed continence rates for YDL at 79%, and 75% for Kropp and Pippi-Salle repairs. Another retrospective review involved 18 children who underwent a Pippi-Salle reconstruction with neurogenic incontinence and showed a dry rate (4 hours or more between catheterizations) of 61%.[8] One of the few prospective studies by Snodgrass and Barber[9] compared initial and long-term continence in 37 consecutive patients with neurogenic bladder undergoing LM plus a BNS with 34 previous consecutive patients undergoing sling alone. The cohorts were equivalent with regard to gender, ambulatory status, and preoperative urodynamic parameters. Initial continence (dry, no pads) determined at 6 months after surgery was significantly different: 29 (78%) of 37 in the LM reconstruction with sling versus 18 (53%) of 34 with sling alone (P = .04). Kaplan-Meier curves showed initially dry sling patients to have recurrent incontinence during follow-up, leaving fewer than 25% dry long term,

versus no loss of continence in LM plus sling patients after 18 months, with 60% still dry at maximum follow-up of 55 months. As can be seen, in spite of the multiple limitations, studies reviewing these BNR techniques report reasonable continence rates ranging from 50% to 85%.[10]

Bladder Neck Closure

Perhaps the most radical option for achieving continence is closure of the bladder neck. A retrospective review by Bergman and colleagues[5] included 52 patients with mixed etiology incontinence undergoing bladder neck closure as primary surgery after failed medical therapy and showed an 88% dry rate. Another study by Liard and colleagues[11] involving 21 patients with bladder neck closure as primary surgical therapy showed an 80% dry rate. Finally, another retrospective study by Hoebeke and colleagues[12] in 17 children undergoing bladder neck closure showed a dry rate of 100% but difficulty with catheterization in 47% of patients.

Laparoendoscopic Procedures for Urinary Continence

Bladder neck injection

A brief analysis of bladder neck injections for outlet incompetence and incontinence makes it clear that the success rates for this modality are extremely low. For example, Lotmann and colleagues[13] performed a prospective trial using Deflux (Salix Pharmaceuticals, Inc., Raleigh, NC, USA) at the bladder neck in 27 children with neurogenic bladder (4 after failed sling). With a mean follow-up of 26 months, they describe a 30% dry rate. Similarly, a retrospective evaluation in 27 patients with persistent outlet incompetency after fascial sling who then underwent injection with either Deflux (3) or Macroplastique (Uroplasty, Inc., Minnetonka, MN, USA) (24) showed a dry rate of 7%, and repeat injections did not improve outcomes.[14] Essentially no study using endoscopic injection at the bladder neck regardless of volume used or injection technique has shown a success rate higher than 33%.[15]

Robotic-Assisted Bladder Neck Reconstruction

Establishing urinary continence in pediatric patients with sphincteric incompetence usually involves a combination of medical therapy, CIC, and sometimes surgical intervention. This condition is most often encountered in children with spina bifida, and is diagnosed by persistent incontinence despite CIC and anticholinergics in patients with detrusor areflexia and detrusor leak point pressure less than 50 cm H2O on urodynamic testing. Cystography demonstrates a smooth-walled bladder and, typically, an open bladder neck. The most commonly used procedure to gain continence in these patients is BNS. However, our data indicate that an LM BNR to reduce the caliber of the outlet, plus sling (LMS) has higher continence rates than a sling alone.[16] Consequently, we perform this procedure and APV (or Monti channel when the appendix is inadequate) to achieve urinary continence in this patient population using robotic assistance. Whether or not an augmentation ileocystoplasty should be concomitantly performed is beyond the scope of this article, but the techniques described later in this article can be implemented and easily modified to accommodate an augmentation when indicated.

It is clear from our data (see later in this article) that the robotic approach offers the same continence for an LMS with the added advantages of small "band aid" incisions, less postoperative pain, and shorter hospitalization. We now almost exclusively do these operations robotically at our institution. We have previously reported our initial results[3] and provide our technique and outcomes.

DESCRIPTION OF TECHNIQUE

The following is the step-by-step description of the technique for a robotic-assisted BNS with BNR (LM) and an APV. Given the excellent exposure to the pelvis and the bladder, this technique can be modified to accommodate any type of bladder neck repair (eg, Salle, Kropp, Young-Dees) (Appendix).

Patient Positioning

The child is placed supine on a padded bean-bag patient positioner (**Fig. 1**). Alternatively, the legs can be placed in lithotomy stirrups. It is imperative to pad all pressure points, including the heels (**Fig. 2**). The patient is secured to the bed using wide tape. The shorter end of the base of the operating room (OR) table should be oriented toward the patient's feet to allow as much space as possible for the base of the robot (**Fig. 3**). Along these lines, the patient should be moved down on the operating table as much as possible. The patient is prepped and draped. The head of the operating table is lowered (Trendelenburg position) for the bladder neck portion of the surgery. A Foley catheter is inserted transurethrally and the balloon inflated to later help identify the bladder neck. This is done sterile on the field. Before positioning, it is recommended (especially early in the surgeon's experience) to cystoscopically place externalized ureteral catheters to aid in ureteral orifice identification during the BNR.

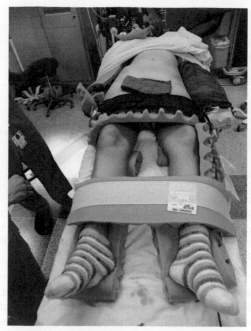

Fig. 1. Patient positioning. It is imperative to meticulously pad every possible pressure point. Alternatively, the patient can be placed in lithotomy, although we do not recommend it, given the potential for lower extremity nerve injury during long cases.

They are secured to the Foley and prepped onto the field.

Skin Incision and Port Placement

An inverted "V"-shaped incision is made in the umbilicus with the apex of the "V" at the base of the umbilicus. The umbilical stalk is grasped with a Kocher clamp and access is obtained with a Veress needle technique. A 5-mm VersaStep (Covidien, Mansfield, MA, USA) trocar is placed and a 5-mm laparoscopic camera is used to place the remaining ports. Port placement is as shown in **Fig. 4**. The robotic ports are secured to the

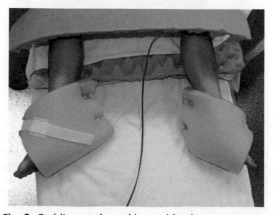

Fig. 2. Padding at the ankles and heels.

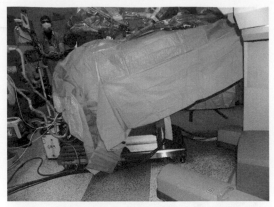

Fig. 3. Docking. The shorter end of the base of the OR table should be oriented toward the patient's feet to allow as much space as possible for the base of the robot.

patient's skin as shown in **Fig. 5** using two 0.5-inch Steri-Strips which are wrapped around the trocar and a small Tegaderm adhesive dressing is used to secure them to the skin. A 2-0 Vicryl suture on a UR6 needle is then used to secure the dressing to the skin and deep subcutaneous tissues. These sutures are then wrapped around the 8.5-mm trocars.

Dissection of the Appendix

Before the robot is docked, the entire right and mid transverse colon are mobilized laparoscopically to

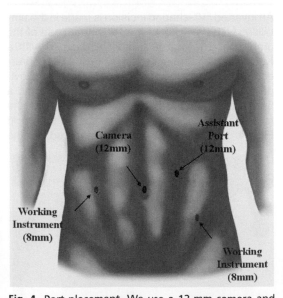

Fig. 4. Port placement. We use a 12-mm camera and two 8.5 working ports. If any bowel work is going to be performed or if a sling is going to be used we use a 12-mm assist in the left upper quadrant. If just an APV is going to be performed, a 5-mm assist port can be used.

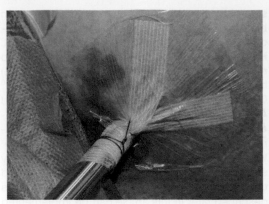

Fig. 5. The robotic ports are secured to the patient's skin as shown using two 0.5-inch Steri-Strips that are wrapped around the trocar and a small Tegaderm adhesive dressing is used to secure them to the skin. A 2-0 Vicryl suture on a UR6 needle is then used to secure the dressing to the skin and deep subcutaneous tissues. These sutures are then wrapped around the 8.5-mm trocars. (3M, St. Paul, MN.)

allow for the appendix to be dissected as inferiorly in the pelvis as possible. The appendix is harvested with a 12-mm laparoscopic Endo-GIA stapler. A cecal extension of the stable line can be used at this point and is particularly helpful in obese patients or in patients with a short appendix.

Robotic Docking

The da Vinci robot (Intuitive Surgical, Inc., Sunnyvale, CA, USA) is docked either directly in the midline from inferior (if the patient is in lithotomy) or slightly from the patient's right side and inferior (**Fig. 6**). The second position allows the surgeon a bit more flexibility to work above the pelvis and to

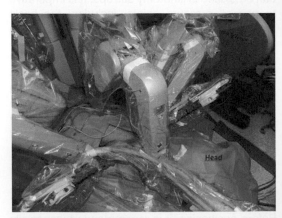

Fig. 6. The Da Vinci robot is docked either directly in the midline from inferior (if the patient is in lithotomy) or slightly from the patient's right side and inferior. (Intuitive Surgical, Sunnyvale, CA.)

the right of the patient in cases in which the appendix needs to be further mobilized. In the second method, the base of the robot should straddle the right corner of the operating table (see **Fig. 3**). Ports are secured to the robotic arms. A 12-mm camera at the 30° up position is used.

Bladder Neck Reconstruction and Sling Placement

Camera: 30° up
Working Instruments:
Right Arm: Monopolar cautery scissors
Left Arm: Robotic DeBakey (Intuitive Surgical, Inc.) or bipolar Maryland

The plane between the vagina and posterior bladder in female patients or the rectum and posterior bladder in male patients is developed. The peritoneum between these structures is opened using a wide horizontal incision. The assistant grasps the inferior lip of this incision and retracts toward themselves (back and down). This plane is dissected as distal as possible. Movement of the Foley and visualization of the balloon can help identify where the end of the bladder neck is. Care must be taken to identify and preserve the vas deferens bilaterally in male patients. Care also must be taken to not carry the dissection too laterally, as this risks potential injury to the ureters. Once this dissection is complete, a second incision is made above the bladder to release the peritoneum, the urachus, and the lateral bladder attachments. This dissection is carried all the way to the lateral pelvic floor, at which point the endopelvic fascia is incised bilaterally and the pubo-prostatic ligaments (in male patients) are released. In adolescent male patients, a dorsal vein suture (2-0 or 3-0 Vicryl) is placed for hemostasis.

Extracorporeal Preparation of the Sling

The sling material preferred is a Suspend-Tutoplast Processed Fascia Lata sling (2 × 7 cm) (Coloplast, Minneapolis, MN, USA). The sling is prepared according with the manufacturer's instructions. Two 12-Fr central line introducers cut at 3 cm are then sewn to each end of the sling. Three air knots are made to create 3 loops between the introducer and the sling. This facilitates retraction by the bedside assistant in the subsequent sections.

Retrovesical Placement of the Sling

Camera: 30° down
Working Instruments:
Right Arm: bipolar Maryland

Left Arm: Monopolar cautery scissors or DeBakey forceps

The sling is passed intracorporeally through the assist port, if 12 mm, if not through one of the 8.5-mm robotic working ports. The attached introducers are placed behind the bladder. One at a time, each introducer is grasped with the Maryland and the space of Retzius is entered bilaterally (**Fig. 7**A, B). Alternatively, this plane can be developed with the bipolar Maryland and once the plane is developed the introducers can be passed anteriorly. At this point, both sides of the sling are passed (see **Fig. 7**C).

Leadbetter/Mitchell Bladder Neck Revision

Camera: 30° down
Working Instruments:
Right Arm: Monopolar cautery scissors
Left Arm: DeBakey forceps

The assistant grasps the loops of suture placed on each end of the sling and retracts cephalad and down. The urethra is incised from 3 to 9 o'clock using the monopolar scissor. The incision is deepened until the urethral catheter and the ureteral stents (if placed) are exposed. The transverse incision is grasped with the left hand and retracted cephalad. The urethra and bladder neck are "unroofed" by carrying the 3 and 9 o'clock incisions in parallel fashion, ending just below the trigone (see **Fig. 7**D). The ureteral orifices can be identified by the previously placed ureteral catheters or by having the anesthesiologist give the patient intravenous indigo carmine. Continuous traction on the midline of the urethra cephalad helps keep the incisions in the same plane, exposing a strip of dorsal urethra, as seen in **Fig. 7**D.

For the tubularization of the bladder neck:
Camera: 30° down
Working Instruments:
Right Arm: Da Vinci black diamond microforceps
Left Arm: Da Vinci black diamond microforceps

A 5-Fr feeding tube is placed into the distal urethra and then the urethra is re-tubularized using 2 layers of continuous, submucosal 4-0 Vicryl then 3-0 Vicryl stitches from distally to proximally (see **Fig. 7**E). It is important to suture close to the edge of the urethral strip, especially through the bladder neck, to ensure the lumen remains uniform in caliber. The feeding tube is left in place and secured to the foreskin or labia minora with a 4-0 silk suture.

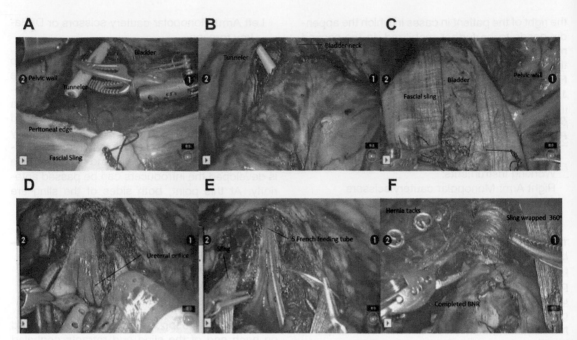

Fig. 7. Steps in the BNR. The tunnelers are passed ventrally from the posterior bladder dissection into the developed space of Retzius (*A, B*). Once the sling is passed from posterior to anterior (*C*), the urethra is unroofed up through the bladder neck to the level of the interureteric ridge (*D*). At this point, the Foley catheter is exchanged for a 5-F feeding tube, and the urethra is retubularized in 2 layers with a running simple suture of 4-0 Vicryl followed by 3-0 Vicryl (*E*). After the LM repair is completed, the sling is tightly wrapped 360° and attached to the pubic bone using 6 screws from a hernia tacker (*F*).

Sling Placement

Right Arm: bipolar Maryland
Left Arm: DeBakey forceps

The central line introducers attached to the sling are detached from the sling and removed. The Maryland on the right arm is passed behind the sling and behind the bladder and the sling end on the patient's right is passed to the Maryland with the left arm (DeBakey forceps). The sling is thus wrapped 360°. The sling is cinched tight.

Right Arm: Da Vinci black diamond microforceps
Left Arm: Da Vinci black diamond microforceps

The sling is secured to itself using 2 interrupted 5-0 Prolene sutures. The ends of the sling are lifted up to the pubic bone. The assistant passes a hernia Tacker Fixation Device (Covidien) and tacks the sling to the pubis using 2 or 3 titanium spiral screws (see **Fig. 7**F).

Bladder Hitch

Camera: 30° down
Working Instruments:
Right Arm: DeBakey forceps
Left Arm: DeBakey forceps

The bladder is hitched to the anterior abdominal wall using 3 interrupted 3-0 polydioxanone (PDS) sutures passed through the abdominal wall or secured intracorporeally. The purpose of this is to bring the bladder as close to the umbilicus and as cephalad as possible and thus minimize the tension on the appendico-vesical anastomosis. If the hitch stitches are passed through the abdominal wall, it is helpful to pass them through a 14-G Angiocath. The hitch stitches are not tied down until the end of the case after the robot is undocked. They are secured at the skin surface using hemostats.

Appendicovesicostomy

Working Instruments:
Right Arm: DeBakey forceps followed by monopolar scissors
Left Arm: DeBakey forceps

The staple line is removed and the tip of the appendix is cut. A 10-Fr feeding tube cut at 10 cm is passed from proximal to distal and the tube is suture ligated to the cecal end of the appendix with a 3-0 PDs suture cut to 10 cm. This allows the tube to be manipulated instead of the appendix. A 4-cm detrusor tunnel is fashioned on the posterior aspect of the bladder.

Appendico-Vesical Anastomosis

Right Arm: Da Vinci black diamond microforceps
Left Arm: Da Vinci black diamond microforceps

A mucosal opening is made on the inferior apex of the detrusor tunnel. The distal end of the appendix is anastomosed using 2 running simple sutures of 5-0 Vicryl on TF needles one up each side.

Detrusor Closure

Right Arm: DeBakey forceps or large needle driver
Left Arm: DeBakey forceps

The detrusor tunnel is closed over the appendix using a running simple 3-0 V-lock suture with a Lapra-Ty at the looped end of the suture. Every-other throw incorporates adventitia on the appendix.

Maturing Stoma

The robot is undocked. The 5-mm laparoscopic camera is turned back on. A Maryland or bowel grasper is passed through the umbilical trocar, the tube sutured to the appendix is grasped, and the appendix is delivered through the umbilical stoma. The appendix is secured to the fascia using a single 4-0 PDS. The appendix is spatulated and the stoma is matured circumferentially to the skin using interrupted 5-0 Vicryl sutures. The 10-Fr feeding tube is exchanged for a 12-Fr or 14-Fr mentor catheter. The mentor catheter is secured to the skin using a 3-0 nylon suture.

Port Closure

All ports are removed and the fascia closed with 2-0 Vicryl on UR6 needles. Skin is closed with 5-0 Monocryl. Dermabond skin adhesive is used. Dressings are optional. All tubes are secured to the skin and attached to drainage bags.

RESULTS

We have now performed 38 robotic-assisted LMS and APVs at our institution and have a mean follow-up of 21 months (range 5–33 months). One of these patients had previously undergone an appendectomy and therefore had a robotic Monti channel created. The male:female ratio is 16%:22% and 90% of these patients had myelomeningocele and neurogenic bladder. Mean patient age was 10 years (range 5–16 years) and mean body mass index was 22.3 (16–31). The mean preoperative bladder capacity was 206 mL (162–308 mL). None of our

patients had previous or simultaneous augmentation. Mean operative time was 5.8 hours (3.6–12.25 hours) with the longer operative times being significantly higher in the first 10 versus the last 28 cases ($P = .0001$). In 4 cases, conversion to open surgery was necessary, because of extensive intra-abdominal adhesions in 2 and an appendix that was not sufficient for APV and so required Monti in 2. Mean hospital length of stay was 52 hours (34–86 hours).

Of the patients, 31 (82%) of 38 are completely dry during the day on CIC every 3 hours. Of the 7 who are wet, 4 are noncompliant with CIC. One is wet from his urethra and Monti channel and 2 developed decreased bladder compliance that was unresponsive to increased anticholinergics and Botox injection, and so underwent ileocystoplasty. Additional complications include 4 cases of de novo reflux (grades 2 and 3), and 2 patients who developed bladder stones. **Fig. 8** shows the postoperative appearance at 6 months.

TIPS AND TRICKS

Robotic-assisted BNR with creation of a continent catheterizable conduit should be considered an "advanced" robotic procedure, and we strongly recommend that surgeons become very familiar and facile with robotic-assisted pyeloplasty and ureteral reimplant before attempting these cases. The following tips and tricks have helped reduce operative time significantly:

- We strongly advise that all the ports be secured to the patient's skin by using a device similar to that shown in **Fig. 5**. Accidental removal of the ports during instrument and robotic arm manipulation can add a significant amount of time to the procedure.
- Mobilization of the entire right and mid transverse colon should be done using free-hand

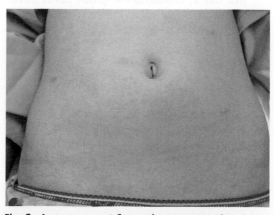

Fig. 8. Appearance at 6 months postoperative.

laparoscopy before docking the robot. Once the robot is docked, it is not possible for the console surgeon to "look" cephalad and, thus, mobilization of the large bowel (if needed to decrease tension of the appendix to bladder anastomosis) is not possible.

- The ideal initial patient should be prepubertal and a female where there is no concern for the vas deferens during the dissection for the sling. We also strongly recommend that the first patient not have a shunt or at least have minimal VP shunt revisions at the abdominal level. VP shunts (especially if they have been revised) cause significant intra-abdominal adhesions, which can make the procedure longer and can contribute to a higher conversion rate (Gargollo and colleagues, manuscript in preparation).
- Management of the VP shunt is controversial. Some investigators advocate placing it in a sterile laparoscopic specimen bag.[17] Until recently, we had had no VP shunt infections without any specific treatment for the shunt. We recently had a cerebrospinal fluid pseudocyst form that required shunt externalization.
- We do not routinely perform a bowel prep for these patients, although some have advocated it to reduce the overall fecal load, especially in patients with neurogenic bowel.
- Using a dorsal venous ligating suture before bladder neck reduction significantly increases visibility.
- All detrusor tunnels were created on the posterior bladder wall because decreased stone formation, urinary tract infection, and increased mucus removal are cited with posterior placement.[18] Maneuvers for improving the operation will surely continue to come to light. The benefits of robot-assisted surgery were evident in most of our patients. Three of 4 patients were discharged on postoperative day 2. Unilateral low-grade reflux developed in 2 patients; it has responded to increased anticholinergic dose.

SUMMARY

In addition to potential for decreased postoperative pain, rapid convalescence, and improved cosmesis, RALS surgery has immense potential with respect to the type of surgery that can be performed in the deep pelvis in children, one of the main reasons this technology has taken a strong foothold in urologic and gynecologic surgery. Because we can achieve the equivalent continence results with the added benefits of smaller incisions, less intraoperative blood loss, less postoperative pain, and shorter hospital stays using robotic assistance as compared with open surgery, we rarely perform open BNR for children with bladder outlet incompetency at our institution. Early in the surgical experience, the surgeon should expect significantly longer operative times when using robotic assistance. However, over time, operative times become significantly shorter and more similar to the duration expected for traditional open surgery for these procedures. Although we perform the LM technique for our bladder neck repairs based on analysis of our outcomes in open surgery, other bladder neck repair techniques also could be adapted to be done robotically. Regardless, when learning such procedures, we recommend the initial patients be thin and prepubertal without previous abdominal surgery, and especially without a ventriculoperitoneal shunt.

Our series is the largest to date reporting complex robotic-assisted lower urinary tract reconstruction for urinary continence. Our data support that these procedures are safe, feasible, and achieve equivalent continence outcomes to open repairs, while providing the additional benefits of shorter hospitalizations and decreased pain. A prospective analysis comparing these methods to open methods is ongoing.

REFERENCES

1. Gundeti MS. Robotic-assisted laparoscopic reconstructive surgery in the lower urinary tract. Curr Urol Rep 2013;14(4):333–41.
2. Gundeti MS. Paediatric robotic-assisted laparoscopic augmentation ileocystoplasty and Mitrofanoff appendicovesicostomy (RALIMA): feasibility of and initial experience with the University of Chicago technique. BJU Int 2011;107(6):962–9.
3. Bagrodia A, Gargollo P. Robot-assisted bladder neck reconstruction, bladder neck sling, and appendicovesicostomy in children: description of technique and initial results. J Endourol 2011;25(8):1299–305.
4. Abrams P. The standardisation of terminology of lower urinary tract function: report from the Standardisation Sub-committee of the International Continence Society. Neurourol Urodyn 2002; 21(2):167–78.
5. Bergman J, Lerman SE, Kristo B, et al. Outcomes of bladder neck closure for intractable urinary incontinence in patients with neurogenic bladders. J Pediatr Urol 2006;2(6):528–33.
6. Dave S, Salle JL. Current status of bladder neck reconstruction. Curr Opin Urol 2008;18(4):419–24.
7. Cole EE, Adams MC, Brock JW 3rd, et al. Outcome of continence procedures in the pediatric patient: a single institutional experience. J Urol 2003;170(2 Pt 1): 560–3 [discussion: 563].

8. Jawaheer G, Rangecroft L. The Pippi Salle procedure for neurogenic urinary incontinence in childhood: a three-year experience. Eur J Pediatr Surg 1999;9(Suppl 1):9–11.

9. Snodgrass W, Barber T. Comparison of bladder outlet procedures without augmentation in children with neurogenic incontinence. J Urol 2010;184(4 Suppl):1775–80.

10. Kropp KA. Bladder neck reconstruction in children. Urol Clin North Am 1999;26(3):661–72, viii.

11. Liard A. The Mitrofanoff procedure: 20 years later. J Urol 2001;165(6 Pt 2):2394–8.

12. Hoebeke P, De Kuyper P, Goeminne H, et al. Bladder neck closure for treating pediatric incontinence. Eur Urol 2000;38(4):453–6.

13. Lottmann HB. Long-term effects of dextranomer endoscopic injections for the treatment of urinary incontinence: an update of a prospective study of 61 patients. J Urol 2006;176(4 Pt 2):1762–6.

14. De Vocht TF. Long-term results of bulking agent injection for persistent incontinence in cases of neurogenic bladder dysfunction. J Urol 2010; 183(2):719–23.

15. DaJusta D, Gargollo P, Snodgrass W. Dextranomer/hyaluronic acid bladder neck injection for persistent outlet incompetency after sling procedures in children with neurogenic urinary incontinence. J Pediatr Urol 2013;9(3):278–82.

16. Snodgrass WT, Gargollo PC. Urologic care of the neurogenic bladder in children. Urol Clin North Am 2010;37(2):207–14.

17. Marchetti P. Management of the ventriculo-peritoneal shunt in pediatric patients during robot-assisted laparoscopic urologic procedures. J Endourol 2011;25(2): 225–9.

18. Berkowitz J. Mitrofanoff continent catheterizable conduits: top down or bottom up? J Pediatr Urol 2009;5(2):122–5.

APPENDIX 1: EQUIPMENT LIST
Robotic-assisted BNR with APV

1. Patient Positioning
   a. Bean-bag positioner
   b. Foam padding
      i. Heel foam wraps
   c. Lithotomy stirrups (optional)
   d. Wide silk tape
   e. Foley catheter (8 or 10 Fr)
   f. Open-ended ureteral stents (4 Fr) (optional)
   g. Laparoscopic drape (optional)
2. Skin Incision and Port Placement
   a. Veress Needle
      i. 5-mm VersaStep trocar
   b. 8.5-mm robotic working trocars ×2 (see figure 4)
      i. 0.5-inch Steri-Strips
      ii. Tegaderm
   c. 5-mm or 12-mm assist port
3. Dissection of the Appendix
   a. Laparoscopic bowel grasper
   b. Harmonic scalpel (optional)
   c. Hook cautery (optional)
   d. Monopolar laparoscopic scissors (optional)
   e. 12-mm laparoscopic Endo-GIA stapler
4. BNR and Sling Placement
   a. 12-mm camera with 30° lens
   b. Da Vinci Monopolar cautery scissors
   c. Da Vinci DeBakey forceps or Da Vinci bipolar Maryland
5. Extracorporeal Preparation of the Sling
   a. Suspend: Tutoplast Processed Fascia Lata sling (2 × 7 cm) (Coloplast)
   b. 2×, 3-0 PDS sutures on RB-1 needles
   c. 2×, 12-Fr central line introducers cut at 3 cm
6. Retrovesical Placement of the Sling
   a. 12-mm camera with 30° lens
   b. Da Vinci Monopolar cautery scissors
   c. Da Vinci DeBakey forceps or Da Vinci bipolar Maryland
7. L/M BNR
   a. 12-mm camera with 30° lens
   b. Da Vinci monopolar cautery scissors
   c. Da Vinci DeBakey forceps
   d. 0.5 ampule of indigo carmine (optional)
   e. 4-0 Vicryl RB-1 needle, 15 cm (first layer)
   f. 3-0 Vicryl RB-1 needle, 15 cm (second layer)
   g. 5-Fr feeding tube
   h. 4-0 silk suture
   i. 2× Da Vinci black diamond microforceps
8. Sling Placement
   a. 12-mm camera with 30° lens
   b. Da Vinci DeBakey forceps
   c. Da Vinci bipolar Maryland
   d. 5-0 Prolene RB-1 needle cut at 12 cm
   e. 2× Da Vinci black diamond microforceps
   f. Laparoscopic Tacker Fixation Device (Covidien)
9. Bladder Hitch
   a. 12-mm Camera with 30° lens
   b. Da Vinci DeBakey forceps × 2
   c. 3×, 2-0 PDS sutures on SH needles with the needles straightened out
   d. 14-G Angiocath
   e. 3 curved hemostats
10. APV
   a. 12-mm camera with 30° lens
   b. Da Vinci DeBakey forceps × 2
   c. 10-Fr feeding tube cut at 10 cm
   d. 3-0 PDS suture on RB-1 cut at 10 cm

11. Appendico-Vesical Anastomosis
   a. Black diamond microforceps × 2
   b. 5-0 Vicryl suture on TF needle cut at 12 cm
   c. 5-0 Vicryl suture on TF needle cut at 10 cm
12. Detrusor Closure
   a. Da Vinci DeBakey forceps × 2
   b. 3-0 V-lock suture with Lapra-Ty at the looped end of the suture

13. Maturing Stoma
   a. 4-0 PDS to secure appendix to fascia
   b. 5-0 Vicryl sutures to circumferentially mature stoma
   c. 12-Fr or 14-Fr mentor catheter
   d. 3-0 nylon suture to secure catheter
14. Port Closure
   a. 2-0 Vicryl on UR-6 needle
   b. 5-0 Monocryl

The Robotic Appendicovesicostomy and Bladder Augmentation
The Next Frontier in Robotics, Are we There?

Andrew J. Cohen, MD*, Joseph J. Pariser, MD, Blake B. Anderson, MD,
Shane M. Pearce, MD, Mohan S. Gundeti, MB, MCh, FEBU, FRCS (Urol), FEAPU

KEYWORDS

- Robotics • Bladder augmentation • Neurogenic bladder • Continent • Mitrofanoff
- Minimally-invasive

KEY POINTS

- Surgeons are gaining robotic experience from pyeloplasty and ureteral reimplantation, and are now performing more complex pediatric cases robotically, such as augmentation ileocystoplasty and Mitrofanoff appendicovesicostomy.
- Data from early case series demonstrate adequate safety and efficacy with outcomes and complication rates similar to those of open techniques.
- The benefits of robotic surgery, including decreased pain, decreased length of stay in hospital, and improved cosmesis, must be balanced with the learning curve, cost, and operative time.

INTRODUCTION

Robotic techniques are being increasingly used in minimally invasive pediatric urology.[1] Pediatric surgeons have gained experience with robotic procedures in children, and are beginning to apply these techniques in more complex cases, such as robotic-assisted laparoscopic augmentation ileocystoplasty and Mitrofanoff appendicovesicostomy (RALIMA). Historically, ileocystoplasty and Mitrofanoff appendicovesicostomy (IMA) have been performed as an open procedure, but a robotic approach in children yields the benefits of minimally invasive surgery; this includes decreased incisional pain, shorter length of stay in hospital, and improved cosmesis.[2]

Laparoscopic-assisted appendicovesicostomy was first described in 1993.[3] That procedure involved laparoscopic mobilization of the colon and appendix followed by implantation of the appendix in the bladder using a lower abdomen incision. Evolution of the technique eventually resulted in the first completely laparoscopic Mitrofanoff appendicovesicostomy, reported in 2004. These investigators describe the use of carbon dioxide pneumovesicum to achieve bladder wall distension, which facilitated creation of an extravesical detrusor trough and appendicovesical anastomosis.[4]

The first robotic-assisted laparoscopic appendicovesicostomy was performed in 2004, and the first completely intracorporeal RALIMA was reported in 2008.[5,6] Several challenges have hindered the wide application of these complex techniques in pediatric urology, including historical preference for open techniques in children, a lack

Pediatric Urology, Section of Urology, The University of Chicago Medical Center and Comer Children's Hospital, 5841 South Maryland Avenue, MC6038, Chicago, IL 60637, USA
* Corresponding author.
E-mail address: Andrew.Cohen@uchospitals.edu

Urol Clin N Am 42 (2015) 121–130
http://dx.doi.org/10.1016/j.ucl.2014.09.009

of standardized training in pediatric robotic surgery, and inherently smaller working spaces in children. Despite these obstacles, pediatric robotic surgery has advanced to become more widely used, even in infant populations.[7,8] Although the open approach for IMA remains the most common technique, RALIMA has established itself as a viable option for pediatric urologists with considerable robotic expertise. This article presents a detailed review of RALIMA, including a discussion of indications, techniques, technical considerations, outcomes, and future directions.

INDICATIONS AND CONTRAINDICATIONS

Bladder augmentation is indicated in disease states that impair bladder function, often through diminished bladder capacity, and/or reduced compliance associated with high-pressure voiding.[9] Potential underlying abnormalities that affect bladder function include spina bifida, neurogenic bladder, nonneurogenic bladder, bladder exstrophy, prune belly syndrome, and posterior urethral valves.[2,10] Ileocystoplasty increases bladder capacity, improves compliance, and reduces voiding pressures, thus protecting against renal deterioration and improving continence.[11] Mitrofanoff appendicovesicostomy simplifies and facilitates clean intermittent catheterization (CIC). In many patients, CIC via the urethra becomes difficult or impossible because of discomfort, trauma, urethral stricture disease, disability, or noncompliance.

Patient selection is critical when considering bladder augmentation or creation of a continent catheterizable channel. Especially in young children, considerable preoperative counseling must be given to parents and caregivers before embarking on any procedure. Absolute and relative contraindications to IMA include prior appendectomy, inability to perform catheterization, poor access to caregivers, inflammatory bowel disease, and short or irradiated bowel.[12] Lack of an appendix may lead to a Monti catheterizable channel using ileum, although this is not preferred, as it requires a bowel anastomosis and may be associated with a slightly higher complication rate.[13,14] Significant renal impairment is a controversial relative contraindication to bladder augmentation. A recent study found that bladder augmentation did not appear to accelerate progression of renal insufficiency in a cohort of children with chronic kidney disease and neurogenic bladder.[15] Specific to the robotic approach, prior multiple abdominal surgery and severe kyphoscoliosis may increase the likelihood of conversion to an open procedure, owing to extensive adhesions or inability to achieve adequate pneumoperitoneum.

TECHNICAL CONSIDERATIONS

The surgical technique described herein has been previously published by the authors' institution, which to their knowledge has the largest body of experience with RALIMA to date.[6,7]

Preparation

Patients are not typically given mechanical or oral antibiotic bowel preparation before surgery. Perioperative antibiotics are administered within 1 hour of incision to all patients (typically cefazolin, gentamicin, and metronidazole unless allergies are present). If a ventriculoperitoneal shunt is present, the antibiotic regimen is broadened to include vancomycin.

Positioning and Port Placement

The patient is placed in a low lithotomy position with the arms tucked at the side. Appropriate foam padding of the torso, arms, and legs is applied to prevent injury. Padded foam is used to protect the face from collision with robotic arms. The patient is prepped and draped with a Foley catheter placed on the sterile field. Ports are placed as described in **Fig. 1**. Ports include a 12-mm port for the camera, 2 ports for the robotic arms (5–8 mm), and a 10-mm assistant port in the left upper quadrant port to pass sutures and

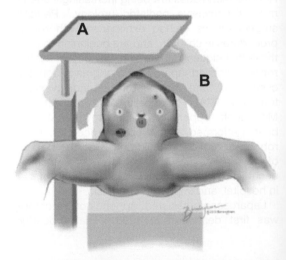

Fig. 1. Port placement and patient positioning. The technique has been modified to no longer use a Mayo stand for facial coverage. (*From* Wille MA, Zagaja GP, Shalhav AL, et al. Continence outcomes in patients undergoing robotic assisted laparoscopic Mitrofanoff appendicovesicostomy. J Urol 2011; 185:1440; with permission.)

irrigate. Occasionally an additional 5-mm port is placed in the right lower quadrant, and can be used later for maturation of the stoma if required.[16] The umbilical stoma is typically used for the maturation of stoma. A minimum puboumbilical distance of 10 to 12 cm is maintained for the camera port. A supraumbilical port site can also be used, which can allow access to both the bowels and bladder.

Operative Technique

The initial 12-mm trocar placement is performed using an open Hassan technique. Once pneumoperitoneum is established, diagnostic peritoneoscopy allows identification of the appendix and its length assessment. In general, the appendix should be approximately 5 to 6 cm and capable of accepting a 10F to 12F catheter to be considered adequate. Of note, numerous substitutions have been described in the literature including ureter, fallopian tubes, tubularized bladder, or colonic flaps. However, there are no published reports of such use during a robotic approach.[17] At this point, the additional robotic and assistant ports are placed under direct vision. If a ventriculoperitoneal shunt is present, the end of the shunt can be placed in an Endopouch retrieval bag (Ethicon, Somerville, NJ, USA) to avoid contamination of the shunt with bowel contents.[18] The appendix is mobilized at the appendicular/cecal junction while maintaining its blood supply (**Fig. 2**). The addition

of cecal flap may reduce the future risk of stomal stenosis. This action may be required when limited by appendiceal length or if both appendicovesicostomy and antegrade colonic enema are planned for management of the bladder and bowel.

The appendix is mobilized at the appendicular/ cecal junction while maintaining its blood supply (see **Fig. 2**B). A 3-0 polyglactin purse-string suture is placed at the base of the appendix and the appendix is then separated from the cecum. The purse-string suture is tied and the cecal opening closed in a second layer with the same suture.

The appendiceal mesentery is then mobilized, and the 1-cm segment of the distal appendix is removed to generate an adequate lumen. The mobility of the appendix is evaluated to confirm it will reach from the bladder to the anterior abdominal wall without tension. Further mobilization of the cecum and right colon can be performed to gain additional mobility. If an augmentation cystoplasty is to be performed, the authors have recently modified the steps of the operation to defer implantation of the appendix until after cystotomy. In this way, an intravesical reimplantation is performed, which seems to decrease the required operative time.

If no additional procedure is planned, the anterior bladder wall is chosen as the insertion site for implantation of the appendix (**Fig. 3**). This technique is technically easier than placing the anastomosis on the posterior wall, especially in patients

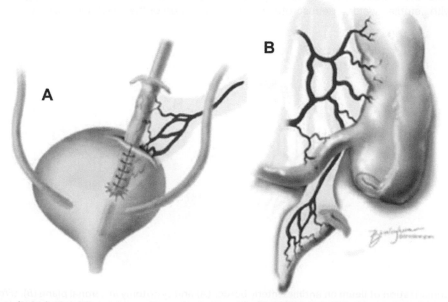

Fig. 2. Appendix isolation (*B*) and appendicovesicostomy with detrusor imbrication on posterior bladder wall (*A*). (*From* Wille MA, Zagaja GP, Shalhav AL, et al. Continence outcomes in patients undergoing robotic assisted laparoscopic Mitrofanoff appendicovesicostomy. J Urol 2011;185:1440; with permission.)

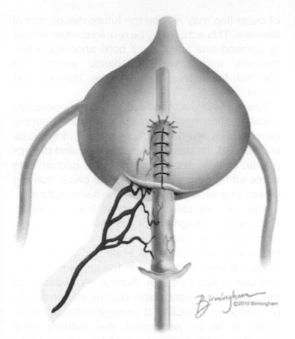

Fig. 3. Placement of appendicovesicostomy on anterior bladder wall. (*From* Wille MA, Zagaja GP, Shalhav AL, et al. Continence outcomes in patients undergoing robotic assisted laparoscopic Mitrofanoff appendicovesicostomy. J Urol 2011;185:1440; with permission.)

with a large bladder.[9] It also shortens the required length of the appendix, as the distance to the abdominal wall is less.

Attention is then turned to implantation of the appendix into the bladder. After distending the bladder with sterile water, detrusorotomy of

approximately 4 cm in length is performed, without entering the mucosa. This action is carried out along the right posterior wall of the bladder if the stoma is matured to skin in the right iliac fossa; otherwise the midline bladder wall is used if creating an umbilical stoma. The first anastomotic suture is placed at the caudalmost apex of the detrusorotomy and then through the spatulated, apical tip of the appendix. The bladder mucosa is incised about 1 cm in length and the appendicovesical anastomosis is completed over an 8F feeding tube. The appendix is next placed in the trough, and the detrusor imbricated over it with a running 4-0 polyglactin suture. A stay suture is placed proximally between the appendix and the proximal extent of the detrusorrhaphy to prevent slippage of the appendix out of the submucosal tunnel. The final appearance is as shown in **Fig. 2**A. In those patients undergoing concomitant cystoplasty, after appendix harvest and the bowel segment for augmentation is isolated, bowel continuity is restored, cystotomy is performed (**Fig. 4**), and the appendix is implanted, followed by detubularized bowel to bladder anastomosis (**Fig. 5**). The authors have previously reported their technique of combined robotic ileocystoplasty and Mitrofanoff appendicovesicostomy.[19]

The proximal end of the appendix is next brought through the umbilical port site or the right lower quadrant through the 8-mm right robotic arm port. Stoma creation is then performed by spatulation of the appendicovesicostomy followed by cutaneous anastomosis using a V flap or a VQZ flap,[20] which provides the advantage of cutaneous coverage of the intestinal mucosa.

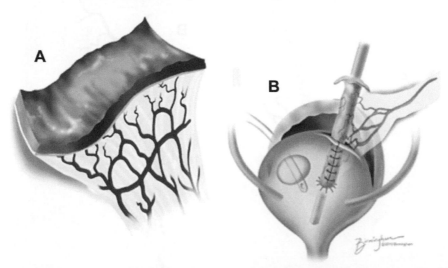

Fig. 4. Detubularization of ileum on antimesenteric border (*A*) and cystotomy in coronal plane (*B*). (*From* Gundeti MS, Acharya SS, Zagaja GP, et al. Pediatric robotic-assisted laparoscopic augmentation ileocystoplasty and Mitrofanoff appendicovesicostomy (RALIMA): feasibility of and initial experience with the University of Chicago technique. BJU Int 2011;107:966; with permission.)

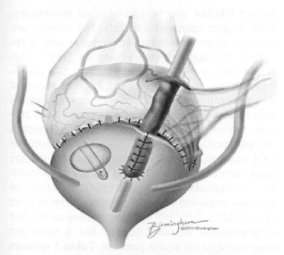

Fig. 5. Completed ileocystoplasty and Mitrofanoff appendicovesicostomy. (*From* Gundeti MS, Acharya SS, Zagaja GP, et al. Pediatric robotic-assisted laparoscopic augmentation ileocystoplasty and Mitrofanoff appendicovesicostomy (RALIMA): feasibility of and initial experience with the University of Chicago technique. BJU Int 2011;107:966; with permission.)

Postoperative Care and Follow-Up

Postoperative care is typical of other minimally invasive surgeries, with goals to minimize narcotics, encourage early diet advancement, and promote ambulation (**Box 1**). In brief, patients are given intravenous ketorolac for 48 hours followed by ibuprofen administration as needed 6 hours after the last dose of ketorolac. A regular diet is started immediately in patients with Mitrofanoff alone, and typically started within 24 hours if undergoing concomitant ileocystoplasty. Patients with baseline constipation are restarted on their home bowel regimen. Discharge criteria include ability to tolerate diet, pain control, and family comfort with drainage tubes.

The appendicovesicostomy and suprapubic catheters are maintained for 4 weeks, at which time the appendicovesicostomy catheter is removed and CIC commences. The suprapubic catheter is capped and maintained as a safety valve for approximately 1 week or until the family is comfortable with CIC. Upper tract evaluation via renal ultrasonography is performed postoperatively.

OUTCOMES AND COMPLICATIONS

Data on outcomes and complications of RALIMA are limited to case series from specialized centers, and it is difficult to directly compare with the gold-standard open approach without case-controlled or randomized trials. Despite these limitations, early outcomes support the safety and efficacy

> **Box 1**
> **Postoperative protocol and follow-up**
>
> *Postoperative Protocol:*
>
> Intravenous ketorolac for 48 hours
>
> Acetaminophen
>
> Regular diet
>
> Home bowel regimen
>
> *Discharge Criteria:*
>
> Tolerates diet
>
> Pain controlled
>
> Comfort with tubes
>
> *Follow-Up:*
>
> Appendicovesicostomy and suprapubic catheter × 4 weeks
>
> Appendicovesicostomy catheter removed and clean intermittent catheterization commences
>
> Suprapubic catheter maintained as safety valve for approximately 1 week
>
> Upper tract evaluation via renal ultrasonography

of RALIMA,[2,9,21,22] with results comparable with those of open series in the literature.[17,23–26]

Important functional outcomes and complications for Mitrofanoff appendicovesicostomy include incontinence, stomal stenosis, stomal prolapse, channel stricture, and false passage formation. In the largest series to date, the authors reported their experience of robotic-assisted Mitrofanoff appendicovesicostomy (RALMA) in 20 patients with a mean follow-up of 24.2 months (range 2.3–43.2 months).[9] Two children were excluded from analysis because they were converted to open surgery owing to adhesions and inadequate appendiceal length. The mean age of the patients was 11 years. Concomitant procedures were performed in 11 (67%) including ileocystoplasty in 10 patients, bladder neck closure, Malone antegrade continence enema, or urethral sling. The mean operative time was 494.1 minutes; however, for those undergoing appendicovesicostomy alone the mean operative time was 323 minutes. The procedure was associated with minimal blood loss and no intraoperative complications. The mean length of stay was 5.2 days. Overall stomal continence rate was 94.4%, and the one child who experienced incontinence within the first year was treated successfully with a single dextranomer/hyaluronic acid injection[27] (Deflux; Salix Pharmaceuticals Inc, Raleigh, NC, USA). Overall, there were 3 stoma-related complications (16.7%) including stomal stenosis in 2 patients and

1 parastomal hernia. Two of these required surgical revision (11.1%). All stoma-related problems were at the skin level; the anastomosis into the bladder remained patent in all.

Two other small series have reported outcomes for RALMA. Nguyen and colleagues[2] published a series of 10 patients who underwent RALMA. Their mean operative time was 323 minutes (range 181–507 minutes). One case was converted to open surgery secondary to inadequate appendiceal length. Mean estimated blood loss was 48.4 mL (range 5–200 mL), median hospitalization was 5 days, and patients were followed up to a median of 14.2 months. Postoperatively, 1 patient required an open revision because of urinary leakage. Minor incontinence developed in 2 cases, of which 1 required dextranomer/hyaluronic acid injection, and 1 resolved without intervention. Storm and colleagues[21] performed robotic appendicovesicostomies in 3 patients with a mean operative time of 301 minutes (range 203–362 minutes). Mean blood loss was 50 mL with a mean hospital stay of 3 days, and patients followed up for 1 to 8 months. All patients were continent, and no complications were reported during the follow-up period.

Pure laparoscopic Mitrofanoff appendicovesicostomy has also been investigated. In a series of 6 children, Nerli and colleagues[22] reported a mean operative time of 139.6 minutes (range 125–175 minutes), mean estimated blood loss of 46 mL, and median length of stay of 7 days. With median follow-up of 33 months, only 2 children developed urinary incontinence, but both responded well to medical therapy. No stomal stenosis or channel strictures were reported.

Review of the literature reveals that complication, continence, and revision rates are similar among RALMA and traditional open techniques. In the largest open series to date, 169 patients underwent open appendicovesicostomy with a reported functional channel rate of 96%. This cohort had a 39% surgical revision rate and a mean follow-up of 5.8 years.[25] Another series of 78 patients who underwent open surgery described a 97% continence rate with a 14% stomal stenosis rate and 23% channel-related complication rate at a mean follow-up of 28.4 months.[17] Additional contemporary groups have reported stomal stenosis as the most common complication from this surgery, with rates of stenosis requiring surgical revision ranging from 16% to 50%.[17,23,24,28–31] Stenosis may be related to inadequate vascular supply, but it does not seem depend on stoma position. **Table 1** reviews outcomes data for both open and robotic series.

Thomas and colleagues[17] reported most stoma-related complications to occur within the first year of surgery, and no complications were identified after 20 months. Welk and colleagues[28] also reported that most channel-related complications developed within the first 2 years of surgery, with a mean follow-up of 28 months. On the other hand, one large review of open surgery identified complications out to 15 years, highlighting the need for continued follow-up for identification of late complications likely caused by change in body habitus and growth.[25]

Ileocystoplasty can lead to additional complications including urinary tract infections, stone formation, metabolic derangements, or renal deterioration. Surer and colleagues[30] reported a 26% incidence of bladder stones in 91 patients with exstrophy-epispadias complex undergoing continent urinary reservoir formation with

Table 1
Selected open and robotic series of Mitrofanoff appendicovesicostomy results

Series	Harris et al[24]	Süzer et al[26]	Thomas et al[17]	Gundeti et al[9]	Nguyen et al[2]
No. of patients	50	36	68	18	10
Technique	Open	Open	Open	Robotic	Robotic
Mean age, y (range)	13.1 (4–25)	10 (3–21)	8.9 (2.5–20)	11 (7–14)	NR (4–18)
Months' follow-up (range)	Mean 13.1 (4–25)	Mean 36 (0.5–78)	Mean 28.4 (6–71)	Median 24.2 (2.3–43.2)	Median 14.2 (3–42.4)
Operative minutes	NR	NR	NR	494.1	323
Mean blood loss, mL (range)	NR	NR	NR	81 (5–400)	48.4 (5–200)
No. stenosis/total no. (%)	5/50 (10)	3/36 (8)	9/68 (13)	3/18 (16)	0/10 (0)
Continence rate (%)	49/50 (98)	NR	66/68 (97)	17/18 (94.4)	9/10 (90)
Revision rate (%)	8/50 (16)	6/36 (17)	9/16 (50)	2/18 (11)	1/10 (10)

Abbreviation: NR, not reported.
Data from Refs.[2,9,17,24,26]

ileocystoplasty. These complications can occur many years after the initial procedure, and have been primarily reported in open series with long-term follow-up.[32,33]

Another concern is the potential for significant adhesions. For children undergoing complex urologic reconstruction there is a potential need for follow-up procedures. In particular, this population has a high incidence of ventriculoperitoneal shunt and may require repeated shunt revisions. The authors previously used a porcine model comparing the postoperative adhesions after robotic versus open ileocystoplasty.[34] The open cohort was found to have significantly more adhesions in terms of number and complexity when assessed by a blinded, third-party surgeon.

The authors also previously compared their experience with robotic and open ileocystoplasty with Mitrofanoff appendicovesicostomy, though in a nonrandomized fashion, and found that while the mean operative time was longer, there was a nonstatistically significant trend toward improved narcotic usage and length of stay (Cohn JA, Murthy P, Dangle PP, et al. Open versus robotic-assisted laparoscopic augmentation ileocystoplasty and Mitrofanoff appendicovesicostomy (RALIMA) for the management of neurogenic bladder in children. 2014. Submitted for publication).

In summary, outcomes and complication data are somewhat limited, as rates have been generally obtained from single-surgeon case series and self-reported events. No current studies directly compare open with robotic approach in a randomized controlled trial. Overall, there does not appear to be an increase in complications associated with RALIMA with follow-up to 24 months. Moreover, both continence and complication rates are similar between minimally invasive and open series. The robotic surgical approach is safe and does not appear to compromise functional outcomes.

CURRENT CONTROVERSIES AND FUTURE CONSIDERATIONS
Current Controversies

The use of robotics has increased in pediatric urology. However, few reports have been published describing experience with pediatric robotic bladder augmentation and/or Mitrofanoff appendicovesicostomy, likely because of the complicated nature of these reconstructive procedures. Some reticence is certainly warranted when using new technology to perform advanced surgical procedures that are relatively uncommon, even in an open setting.

Operative time is a concern when comparing existing literature on these procedures with the traditional open technique. The authors reported a mean operative time of 5.4 hours for 7 children who underwent robotic Mitrofanoff appendicovesicostomy alone, and an overall operative time of 8.2 hours in 18 children in the entire robotic cohort that included many patients who underwent concomitant bladder augmentation and/or other procedures. In the series described by Nguyen and colleagues,[2] 10 patients underwent RALMA with a mean operative time of 5.4 hours. These patients were compared with case-matched historical controls performed in an open fashion, which took a mean of 4.5 hours. However, the investigators argue that their last 3 cases in the cohort averaged 3.7 hours, indicating that after an initial learning curve, a decrease in time should be expected. A similar phenomenon has been reported in the early adoption of robotic technology for other complex urologic procedures, such as radical cystectomy with intracorporeal urinary diversion.[35–37]

There is still some controversy regarding the location of appendicovesicostomy implantation on the bladder wall. Traditionally a posteriorly implanted appendicovesicostomy was performed. However, an anterior approach is technically easier and decreases the appendiceal length needed to reach the abdominal wall, which can be a limiting factor in some children. Some previous reports expressed concern regarding an anteriorly implanted channel with regard to urinary tract infections, mucus clearance, and stone formation. In a retrospective review of an open approach, 33 anteriorly implanted and 21 posteriorly implanted channels were compared. Patients with anterior conduits had an increased risk of bladder stone formation and urinary tract infection, though not statistically significant in the case of stone rates.[38] In the series by Nguyen and colleagues,[2] patients were implanted using both methods, whereas in the authors' series all patients had an anteriorly implanted channel.[9] In these 2 robotic series, bladder stones were not encountered as a complication.

While decreased blood loss and pain are reported benefits of robotic surgery, cost remains a significant concern when considering widespread adoption of robotic technology. The cost of robotics involves the initial purchase of a surgical robot, service contracts, and various disposables. Although no direct cost analyses have been performed in the RALIMA literature, correlates can be found in other realms of robotic urology literature. A systematic review by Ahmed and colleagues[39] in adult urologic surgery concluded that robotics is probably more costly than laparoscopic or open surgery, likely secondary to capital cost, maintenance of the robot, and limited life of the instruments. More specifically to robotic pediatric urology, Seideman and colleagues[40] reported the cost of robotic pyeloplasty to be $10,635, compared with $9065 for laparoscopic pyeloplasty. Another, separate analysis reported the costs of robotic ($15,337) versus laparoscopic ($16,067) pyeloplasty, the results of which were not statistically significant.[41] Of note, these financial analyses are rife with difficulty, owing to the complex and multifaceted institute-dependent factors on cost. Downstream revenue and incentives to the organization at large may negate any higher cost. From the patient's perspective, minimal scars and/or a less invasive surgical option may drive medical decision making and the spending of health care dollars.

Future Directions and Considerations

Widespread adoption of robotic technology has been established for some urologic procedures such as radical prostatectomy. From 2003 to 2010, the use of robotics for radical prostatectomy rose from 0.7% to 42%.[42] Specifically within pediatric urology, initial adoption of robotics has been seen in tertiary centers with the performance of relatively more common procedures such as pyeloplasty or ureteral reimplantation. Large, multicenter, comparative data still are needed in these areas. Few reports exist regarding the use of robotics for more complicated procedures such as bladder augmentation or Mitrofanoff appendicovesicostomy. Although the authors are cautiously optimistic given early positive reports that show results comparable with those of open series, even high-volume centers may only perform 3 to 5 of these cases annually.[43] In addition, the overall number of bladder augmentation procedures has been falling as less invasive procedures such as injection of intravesical botulinum toxin have become more widely used.[11] These factors may also limit the case volume, comfort, and adoption of robotic technology in the treatment of these patients.

Widespread adoption of robotic surgery in pediatric urology would require substantial investments in time, money, and energy in the proper training of residents and fellows. For this technology to be disseminated safely, a robotic curriculum will likely need to be developed. Moreover, trainees would ideally receive accreditation before exploring complex robotic surgeries such as RALIMA in the pediatric population. The case series described herein were performed by expert robotic surgeons with considerable experience with robotically assisted laparoscopic procedures, such as pyeloplasty. Given the associated complexity, length, and steep learning curve, the authors do not advocate rapid adoption of this technique without proper and careful preparation.

The potential development of pediatric-specific robotic components may further influence the field's progression, as much of the current technology in use was specifically designed for adults. Indeed this is an inherent limitation of the present state of robotics, as some maneuvers require creative solutions from the surgical team to overcome technical limitations on robotic arm or instrument movements. Advancements in instrument miniaturization, given the small working space in pediatric patients, may influence future adoption of these techniques.

Telesurgery is one of the future frontiers of surgery in the digital age. Given the use of the robotic console, it is no longer outlandish to imagine a future in which an expert robotic surgeon can operate on a patient remotely. In fact, a remote robot-assisted laparoscopic cholecystectomy was performed in 2002 over a round-trip distance of 14,000 km and only incurred a lag time of 155 milliseconds.[44] In the pediatric population, this may open access globally to patients with complex problems who otherwise would not be able to obtain treatment. Logistic, economic, social, and political obstacles must be overcome before any transcontinental surgery of this type becomes widespread. For now, remote surgery remains a rarity, but it may become more common in our lifetimes.

One of the largest sources of morbidity is in the use of bowel segments and the need for a bowel anastomosis, which increases the convalescent period and complication rate. Tissue engineering remains a promising area of active research that may eventually liberate us from the need to harvest bowel in urologic reconstruction. Atala and colleagues[45] reported the initial clinical experience of augmentation cystoplasty with engineered bladder tissues in 7 patients demonstrating durable improvement in leak-point pressure, capacity, and compliance at a mean follow-up of 46 months. This phase I study used engineered bladder tissue created from autologous cells seeded onto a collagen-based scaffold and wrapped in omentum. Subsequent phase II studies showed less effectiveness using these technologies, with no significant improvements in bladder capacity or compliance.[46] Further research is needed in regenerative medicine to construct durable substitutes for native tissues. The implications of such technology would be widespread across all medical fields, including adult and pediatric urology.

SUMMARY

Robotic surgery is being more widely applied for use in complex pediatric cases, such as RALIMA. Early case reports have demonstrated safety and efficacy, with outcomes and complication rates that compare favorably with those of open techniques. The benefits of minimally invasive surgery include decreased incisional pain, potentially decreased length of stay in hospital, and improved cosmesis. These benefits must be weighed against the steep learning curve, cost, and operative time.

REFERENCES

1. Peters CA. Laparoscopy in pediatric urology. Curr Opin Urol 2004;14:67–73.
2. Nguyen HT, Passerotti CC, Penna FJ, et al. Robotic assisted laparoscopic Mitrofanoff appendicovesicostomy: preliminary experience in a pediatric population. J Urol 2009;182:1528–34.
3. Jordan GH, Winslow BH. Laparoscopically assisted continent catheterizable cutaneous appendicovesicostomy. J Endourol 1993;7:517–20.
4. Hsu TH, Shortliffe LD. Laparoscopic Mitrofanoff appendicovesicostomy. Urology 2004;64:802–4.
5. Pedraza R, Weiser A, Franco I. Laparoscopic appendicovesicostomy (Mitrofanoff procedure) in a child using the da Vinci robotic system. J Urol 2004;171:1652–3.
6. Gundeti MS, Eng MK, Reynolds WS, et al. Pediatric robotic-assisted laparoscopic augmentation ileocystoplasty and Mitrofanoff appendicovesicostomy: complete intracorporeal–initial case report. Urology 2008;72:1144–7 [discussion: 1147].
7. Dangle PP, Kearns J, Anderson B, et al. Outcomes of infants undergoing robot-assisted laparoscopic pyeloplasty compared to open repair. J Urol 2013; 190:2221–6.
8. Kutikov A, Resnick M, Casale P. Laparoscopic pyeloplasty in the infant younger than 6 months–is it technically possible? J Urol 2006;175:1477–9 [discussion: 1479].
9. Famakinwa OJ, Rosen AM, Gundeti MS. Robot-assisted laparoscopic Mitrofanoff appendicovesicostomy technique and outcomes of extravesical and intravesical approaches. Eur Urol 2013;64:831–6.
10. Wille MA, Jayram G, Gundeti MS. Feasibility and early outcomes of robotic-assisted laparoscopic Mitrofanoff appendicovesicostomy in patients with prune belly syndrome. BJU Int 2012;109:125–9.
11. Biers SM, Venn SN, Greenwell TJ. The past, present and future of augmentation cystoplasty. BJU Int 2012;109:1280–93.
12. Khoury JM, Webster GD. Augmentation cystoplasty. World J Urol 1990;8:203–7.
13. Piaggio L, Myers S, Figueroa TE, et al. Influence of type of conduit and site of implantation on the outcome of continent catheterizable channels. J Pediatr Urol 2007;3:230–4.
14. Lemelle JL, Simo AK, Schmitt M. Comparative study of the Yang-Monti channel and appendix for continent diversion in the Mitrofanoff and Malone principles. J Urol 2004;172:1907–10.
15. Ivancić V, Defoor W, Jackson E, et al. Progression of renal insufficiency in children and adolescents with neuropathic bladder is not accelerated by lower urinary tract reconstruction. J Urol 2010;184: 1768–74.
16. Chang C, Steinberg Z, Shah A, et al. Patient positioning and port placement for robot-assisted surgery. J Endourol 2014;28:631–8.
17. Thomas JC, Dietrich MS, Trusler L, et al. Continent catheterizable channels and the timing of their complications. J Urol 2006;176:1816–20 [discussion: 1820].
18. Marchetti P, Razmaria A, Zagaja GP, et al. Management of the ventriculo-peritoneal shunt in pediatric patients during robot-assisted laparoscopic urologic procedures. J Endourol 2011;25:225–9.
19. Gundeti MS, Acharya SS, Zagaja GP, et al. Paediatric robotic-assisted laparoscopic augmentation ileocystoplasty and Mitrofanoff appendicovesicostomy (RALIMA): feasibility of and initial experience with the University of Chicago technique. BJU Int 2011; 107:962–9.
20. Landau EH, Gofrit ON, Cipele H, et al. Superiority of the VQZ over the tubularized skin flap and the umbilicus for continent abdominal stoma in children. J Urol 2008;180:1761–6.
21. Storm DW, Fulmer BR, Sumfest JM. Laparoscopic robot-assisted appendicovesicostomy: an initial experience. J Endourol 2007;21:1015–7.
22. Nerli RB, Reddy M, Devraju S, et al. Laparoscopic Mitrofanoff appendicovesicostomy: our experience in children. Indian J Urol 2012;28:28–31.
23. Liard A, Séguier-Lipszyc E, Mathiot A, et al. The Mitrofanoff procedure: 20 years later. J Urol 2001;165: 2394–8.
24. Harris CF, Cooper CS, Hutcheson JC, et al. Appendicovesicostomy: the Mitrofanoff procedure-a 15-year perspective. J Urol 2000;163:1922–6.
25. Leslie B, Lorenzo AJ, Moore K, et al. Long-term followup and time to event outcome analysis of continent catheterizable channels. J Urol 2011;185: 2298–302.
26. Süzer O, Vates TS, Freedman AL, et al. Results of the Mitrofanoff procedure in urinary tract reconstruction in children. Br J Urol 1997;79:279–82.
27. Wille MA, Zagaja GP, Shalhav AL, et al. Continence outcomes in patients undergoing robotic assisted laparoscopic Mitrofanoff appendicovesicostomy. J Urol 2011;185:1438–43.

28. Welk BK, Afshar K, Rapoport D, et al. Complications of the catheterizable channel following continent urinary diversion: their nature and timing. J Urol 2008; 180:1856–60.

29. Fishwick JE, Gough DC, O'Flynn KJ. The Mitrofanoff procedure: does it last? BJU Int 2000;85:496–7.

30. Surer I, Ferrer FA, Baker LA, et al. Continent urinary diversion and the exstrophy-epispadias complex. J Urol 2003;169:1102–5.

31. Cain MP, Casale AJ, King SJ, et al. Appendicovesicostomy and newer alternatives for the Mitrofanoff procedure: results in the last 100 patients at Riley Children's Hospital. J Urol 1999;162:1749–52.

32. Gurung PM, Attar KH, Abdul-Rahman A, et al. Long-term outcomes of augmentation ileocystoplasty in patients with spinal cord injury: a minimum of 10 years of follow-up. BJU Int 2012;109:1236–42.

33. Johnson EU, Singh G. Long-term outcomes of urinary tract reconstruction in patients with neurogenic urinary tract dysfunction. Indian J Urol 2013; 29:328–37.

34. Razmaria AA, Marchetti PE, Prasad SM, et al. Does robot-assisted laparoscopic ileocystoplasty (RALI) reduce peritoneal adhesions compared with open surgery? BJU Int 2014;113:468–75.

35. Collins JW, Tyritzis S, Nyberg T, et al. Robot-assisted radical cystectomy (RARC) with intracorporeal neobladder—what is the effect of the learning curve on outcomes? BJU Int 2014;113:100–7.

36. Desai M, de Abreu AL, Goh AC, et al. Robotic intracorporeal urinary diversion: technical details to improve time efficiency. J Endourol 2014. [Epub ahead of print].

37. Pruthi RS, Smith A, Wallen EM. Evaluating the learning curve for robot-assisted laparoscopic radical cystectomy. J Endourol 2008;22:2469–74.

38. Berkowitz J, North AC, Tripp R, et al. Mitrofanoff continent catheterizable conduits: top down or bottom up? J Pediatr Urol 2009;5:122–5.

39. Ahmed K, Ibrahim A, Wang TT, et al. Assessing the cost effectiveness of robotics in urological surgery—a systematic review. BJU Int 2012;110:1544–56.

40. Seideman CA, Sleeper JP, Lotan Y. Cost comparison of robot-assisted and laparoscopic pyeloplasty. J Endourol 2012;26:1044–8.

41. Casella DP, Fox JA, Schneck FX, et al. Cost analysis of pediatric robot-assisted and laparoscopic pyeloplasty. J Urol 2013;189:1083–6.

42. Chang SL, Kibel AS, Brooks JD, et al. The impact of robotic surgery on the surgical management of prostate cancer in the United States. BJU Int 2014. [Epub ahead of print].

43. Lendvay TS. Editorial comment. J Urol 2009;182: 1534.

44. Marescaux J, Leroy J, Rubino F, et al. Transcontinental robot-assisted remote telesurgery: feasibility and potential applications. Ann Surg 2002;235: 487–92.

45. Atala A, Bauer SB, Soker S, et al. Tissue-engineered autologous bladders for patients needing cystoplasty. Lancet 2006;367:1241–6.

46. Joseph DB, Borer JG, De Filippo RE, et al. Autologous cell seeded biodegradable scaffold for augmentation cystoplasty: phase II study in children and adolescents with spina bifida. J Urol 2014;191: 1389–95.

MIS-Behavior
Practical Heuristics for Precise Pediatric Minimally Invasive Surgery

Thane A. Blinman, MD

KEYWORDS

• Minimally invasive surgery • Mechanical advantage • Pediatric urology • Pediatrics

KEY POINTS

• Do not confuse flashy technology as a substitute for precision technique, or for knowing how devices were designed to be used.
• Precise movement follows from specific measures that favor the surgeon's mechanical advantage.
• Moving well in MIS is always a two-handed effort, in terms of coordinated motion, tension, visualization, and especially training.
• Precision in pediatric MIS results from a conscious rejection of the kind of movement disallowed in open surgery but often overlooked or excused in MIS.

INTRODUCTION

Minimally invasive surgery (MIS) is hard to teach. To begin with, it is hard to learn.[1,2] Successful MIS originates in good, open surgical technique, but routine surgical skills translate poorly to MIS. The natural habits of humans conflict with the unfamiliar and counterintuitive methods of MIS, hampering application, and sometimes producing rotten results.[3] The job seems even harder in small children. A child half as tall as an adult offers surgical spaces with just one-eighth the volume. Pediatric MIS can seem 8 times as difficult.

Despite skepticism about pediatric MIS,[4,5] benefits are plainly demonstrated.[6,7] Because MIS offers the surgeon and the pediatric patient nontrivial advantages in terms of wounds, infections,[8] information,[9] precision, visualization, and even speed, MIS is here to stay. MIS forms a central part of surgical training, obviating the notion of the MIS fellowship. MIS should be just another part of pediatric general, thoracic, and urologic surgery.

Nevertheless, clumsy laparoscopic technique is anything but "minimally invasive." Perhaps this explains why reports of MIS in children often hedge with a caveat about "in skilled hands" or "in centers with adequate experience."[10] Ad hoc practices and imprecise maneuvers produce long anesthetic times, poor mechanical results,[11] and return trips to the operating room. Only precision MIS lives up to the promise to help better and hurt less.

Unfortunately, typical surgical pedagogy does not prepare residents to be precise. As actually practiced, training often does not consist of transmission of principled, applied methods mastered by deliberate practice. Instead, it consists of residents absorbing surgical memes[12] in monkey-see, monkey-do fashion. Young surgeons who do not grasp the rationale for each move simply ape poor moves poorly. Results suffer, unless luck prevails.

Surgical precision is the single critical route to patient safety in pediatric MIS. Here precision

Division of General, Thoracic and Fetal Surgery, Children's Hospital of Philadelphia, 34th and Civic Center Boulevard, Philadelphia, PA 19104, USA
E-mail address: blinman@email.chop.edu

Urol Clin N Am 42 (2015) 131–140
http://dx.doi.org/10.1016/j.ucl.2014.09.011
0094-0143/15/$ – see front matter © 2015 Elsevier Inc. All rights reserved.

means exact achievement of the desired surgical (mechanical) objective using the most parsimonious motion. However, surgical precision will not emerge from contrived checklists[13] or Likert scales or milestones. A surgeon might rather be lucky than good, but skill creates its own luck.

This article offers some principles of good pediatric MIS technique that can be taught and practiced. These heuristics can improve the surgeon's mechanical advantage for any MIS case, in any size patient. Mechanical advantage (eg, improved torque, increased degrees of freedom) may seem nebulous, but it is always recognized by a peculiar sense of physical relief. The surgeon with mechanical advantage exerts less effort, makes fewer moves, feels less fatigue, and places the needle or hook exactly. Moreover, a good heuristic always contains a real verb, an observable action taking an actual object (institutional verbs do not; eg, optimize, foster, strive, endeavor, assess). Principles should apply in the real world.

TECHNOLOGY IS NOT TECHNIQUE

Tools do not perform the operation. For example, the surgical robot is really a telemanipulator or waldo. Tools cannot make a novice surgeon into an expert, even if hospitals cannot resist using these devices in their advertisements. Devices should be understood as a tool for something. The surgical telemanipulator is a tool for increasing surgical degrees of freedom and for offering better movement than rigid instruments. A stapler is a tool for tissue approximation. However, endoscopic gadgets are rarely designed for very small patients, and trying to force these devices invites error (eg, trying to squeeze a standard endoscopic stapler into an infant's chest). Features easily become bugs when the tools are misunderstood.

On the other hand, the expert surgeon has developed robust and general skills with basic endoscopic instruments. His or her suture technique is as precise as the open technique. He or she can safely and rapidly perform many procedures at least as well as (and, in many cases, better than) using open technique. Use of gadgets fosters shortcuts and poor methods, compromises outcomes, and lends MIS an air of risk. In cases of trouble, the patient is always better served by reliable technique than by technology.

An important corollary here is that the expert knows how all the tools work. She or he knows how the tools are assembled, how feedback is measured, how the various energy sources work, and what the limits and liabilities are. For example, the novice is baffled by insufflation problems. An

expert quickly recognizes a problem and tracks possible causes from the wall to the patient, from the CO_2 source, to the insufflator, to the tubing, to the trocars, to the instruments, to the depth of anesthesia. Similarly, the expert chooses hook, spatula, hot scissors, Harmonic Scalpel (Ethicon, Endosurgery, Cincinnati, OH, USA), or Ligasure (ValleyLab, Boulder, CO, USA) according to a desired tissue effect, how the shape of the business end fits his or her surgical field, and what problems are minimized by choosing one over the other. The novice has a single tool and tries to use it everywhere (eg, trying to use the Harmonic scalpel as a magic coagulator on a liver capsule bleed).

MIS is not technology, but it depends on it. The right tools — camera, ports, instruments, scopes — make the difference between a safe operation performed smoothly under conditions of excellent visualization...and a "flail." The expert surgeon protects patients from the hidden cost-increases that accompany pennywise administrative choices by insisting on tools that offer objective advantages.

Although an experienced surgeon will be irritated by clunky instruments, the novice will be flummoxed, operating with jerky moves and halting over-corrections. The delicate infant liver, fine sutures, and ephemeral tissue planes become casualties of the novice surgeon's distress. Then, disrupted anatomy and bloody views make the operation even harder, producing a feed-forward spiral to suboptimal results at best and disaster at worst. Well-chosen, well-functioning tools must be regarded (and budgeted for) as indispensable contributors to patient safety. A novice blames the tools; the expert's tools serve her or his technique.

A hidden hazard with surgical devices lies in implied uses, sometimes called affordances.[14] Rarely are surgeons given instruction on the elements of devices' designs, and user manuals are an early casualty of a busy operating room. Instead, surgeons in training typically receive casual lessons or lore, often passed from a senior resident, lessons they may pass to their own trainees. Sometimes, those lessons are correct; however, they are often only someone's work-around (eg, a Malecot drain repurposed as a gastrostomy tube). Other times, the use is simply a misunderstanding of a design that implies by its shape or structure that it should be used a particular way.

Sometimes, these hints for use are accurate but, without a real why behind some practice, the novice will have no basis with which to tell. For example, novice operators think they must always insert finger and thumb into laparoscopic instruments, often forcing the hand into awkward supination. The way around this is to palm the instrument, using a light grip.

The surgeon must understand when the design does not quite serve, how these shortcomings can increase risks, and how to mitigate them. For example, some surgical staplers require a relatively strong grip to fire. A surgeon with smaller hands may be at a serious mechanical disadvantage, shaking struggles during firing may translate to risky jarring at the business end. One way around this is to turn the handle upside down, lengthening the effective moment arm (torque = force × moment arm length), decreasing the force required to exert the same torque on the firing mechanism.

Of course, another way around this problem is to use another method. The expert has no problem switching from a stapler to a suture, endoloop, or clip. She or he has mastered multiple methods and so has greater versatility. Expert MIS technique is enabled by technology but not limited to the technology.

SET UP FOR MECHANICAL ADVANTAGE
Face the Organ!

Mechanical advantage requires good patient positioning. However, positioning the patient properly actually begins with positioning the surgeon. Too often, surgeons operate awkwardly, stricken by the paradoxic action of their tools on the screen. Precision movement is laughable when the surgeon cannot intuit right and left, up and down. Of course, it is not funny for the surgeon.

Perfect position allows the surgeon to operate with small effort. The most important principle for good position that the surgeon should face the organ he or she is operating on. In other words, the surgeon should place the monitor in a line with herself or himself, the camera, and the organ of interest. An old mnemonic is S-C-O-P: surgeon → camera → organ → picture. For example, with appendectomy, the surgeon stands to the patient's left, facing the right lower quadrant with the screen on the patient's right. Alternatively, when operating on the gastroesophageal junction, the surgeon should stand at the foot of the bed (with babies frog-legged at the end of the bed, larger patients in low lithotomy position) facing the epigastrium, with the monitor hung directly over the patient's chest (**Fig. 1**).

Meanwhile, poor position exhausts the surgeon. As the surgeon fatigues, the muscles responsible for fine movements fail first,[15] degrading precision. For example, a surgeon who attempts to operate on a spleen from the patient's left not only

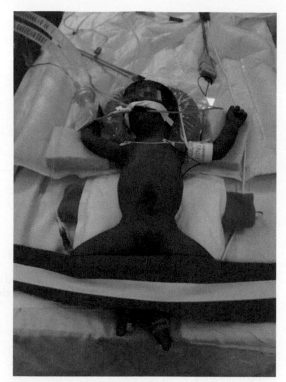

Fig. 1. In small children, facing the organ may place the surgeon in unfamiliar locations, such as at the foot when operating in the upper abdomen (eg, for fundoplication, duodenal atresia repair, or biliary reconstruction). Notice that the baby is well padded and secured, with a warming pad beneath.

struggles with a poor angle of attack and paradoxic motion, but the awkward body position quickly leads to fatigue. If the surgeon is shaking and sore after the procedure, the set-up was probably suboptimal.

Implicit in this rule is knowing what the organ is. For example, when performing a thoracoscopic lobectomy, the organ is not the lung or the lobe; it is the major fissure, the place where most of the fine dissection occurs (**Fig. 2**), and the surgeon should stand in line with it. Similarly, when performing laparoscopic procedures on the infant bladder or rectum the surgeon should stand at the baby's head.

One mental barrier to facing the organ is the implicit rule that a surgeon and an assistant must operate opposite each other (with even left and right sides implying surgical hierarchy). Any other arrangement seems wrong, even taboo. However, what brings advantage in open cases may bring disadvantage in MIS cases. It is absurd for either surgeon or assistant to struggle with paradoxic motion. This unwise practice is tolerated because of the belief that an operator must stand on each

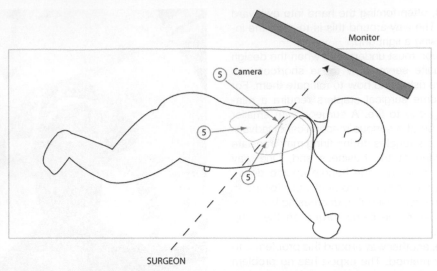

Fig. 2. Proper positioning and trocar placement depend on defining what the organ for a case really is. In this case, the organ is not the lung or lobe, it is the fissure. The circled 5s are 5 mm trocar placements in this infant.

side of the patient regardless of the surgical objective. Facing the organ goes for surgeon and assistant, even if both stand on the same side of a patient (as they often should).

Imitate the Pianist

Only when facing the organ can the other aspect of good positioning be used: the pianist position. Virtuoso pianists hold their arms loose at the shoulder, arms bent at the elbow, wrists loose, and fingers on the keys. Virtuoso endoscopic surgeons operate with the bed at a level that allows them the same position: head upright and level with the screen,[16] shoulders relaxed, elbows bent at 90° to 120°, wrists loose, and action on the instruments controlled with light pressure in the fingertips. The novice can be seen with back bent, arms abducted, elbows askew, wrists stiff, and instruments held in a death grip. Expert surgeons' moves look fluid and relaxed compared with the novice's, in large part because the expert's positioning is better. The comfortable surgeon attends to surgical detail; the uncomfortable surgeon thinks about his or her sore back.

Maximize Degrees of Freedom

Positioning the patient and the surgeon are part of a good set up. Port placement is another. In general, the camera is in the center (however, not always; see later discussion) and trocars should be placed so that right-hand and left-hand instruments approach the organ of interest separated by approximately 90°. Meanwhile, the camera port should be offset from the ? main working

ports such that the 3 ports form a triangle, not a line. These 4 points, the 3 main ports and the organ, form a kite-like shape, a configuration that generally allows the best view, comfort, and maneuverability (**Fig. 3**).

Even in small patients, the kite allows wide enough separation between ports; therefore, the operator will not cross the streams and impede the work. Equal spacing allows both hands to contribute similarly. Even if 4 or more ports are needed, the position of all ports is determined by the working triangle.

The underlying principle here is to maximize the degrees of freedom available to the surgeon. Degrees of freedom refers to the mechanical definition: the number of parameters needed to

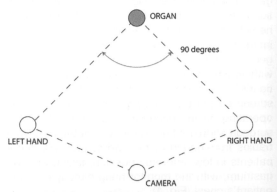

Fig. 3. Trocars should be positioned to maximize the range of degrees of freedom for movement of each working port. This basic kite shape with the object of the operation at the lung apex can be modified (extra ports, the outrigger camera), but the essential aim is to avoid constraining available movement.

describe a body or system in space. For example, a train on a track has a single degree of freedom, its position on the track. In contrast, the human hand has 27 degrees of freedom.[17]

A nonarticulated laparoscopic instrument placed through the body wall has, at most, 6° of freedom:

1. Swinging parallel to the plane of the body wall
2. Moving normal to the plane of the body wall
3. Moving in and out through the port
4. Rotating within the port
5. Motions at the tip (ie, the jaw action)
6. Translation of the body wall plane (ie, as with insufflation, which pushes the abdominal wall upward).

The da Vinci robot adds 2 more degrees of freedom, with 2 directions of articulation at the wrist of the instrument. It does this at a cost of around $2 million. In other words, in MIS a single degree of freedom is worth a million dollars! The surgeon would do well to position the ports (and herself or himself) in such a way that no degree of freedom is restricted or eliminated. For example, surgeons may place the working trocars too far from the organ of interest. The instruments are nearly parallel, and degrees of freedom 1, 2, and 3 are seriously reduced. Similarly, an unrelaxed patient may clamp down on the abdominal wall, overcoming the insufflation pressure, thereby translating the abdominal wall downward. The same effect can be seen with a lazy camera operator who pushes the abdomen down in a baby while driving the camera. This downward translation of the body wall constrains all other motion.

Forbid Paradoxic Motion

Triangulating the ports centers the camera, keeping paradoxic motion to a minimum. Paradoxic motion means attempting to operate when the image is reversed, from the surgeon's perspective. A ready illustration of the awkwardness this creates is experienced simply by turning a computer mouse upside down and trying to move the cursor where necessary. Paradoxic motion happens when the surgeon violates the principle of face the organ. For example if the camera was looking toward the appendix, but the surgeon was standing on the patient's right, he or she would be working paradoxically. All moves would feel backwards and unintuitive. No one can operate with precision this way.

However, rigidly keeping the camera in the center port may be disadvantageous. Occasionally, operations are better performed (at least in part) by placing the camera to one side, as an outrigger

camera. For example, in appendectomy, it may be easier to place the camera at the umbilicus and work through suprapubic and left-lower-quadrant ports. In thoracoscopic diaphragmatic hernia repair with the patient in decubitus position, it may be advantageous to have the camera (and the camera operator) in the port nearest the patient's back and the operator using the ports in the midaxillary and anterior axillary lines. In other cases, the peculiarities of the anatomy (eg, some thoracic masses) may require the camera to occupy any of the ports as the procedure progresses. Triangulating the ports allows the freedom to move the camera whenever needed, without creating distortions in working mechanical advantage. In each of these cases, using an angled scope allows an outrigger camera to minimize paradoxic motion.

Use Gravity Like Another Assistant

Using gravity can dramatically improve visibility, decrease the need for manipulating the organs, and cut anesthetic time. For example, when operating in the pelvis, the worst possible position would be reverse-Trendelenburg; all of the small bowel would slide to the pelvis, hopelessly obscuring all other structures. On the other hand, when operating in the upper quadrants, especially, for example, during a fundoplasty or a gastric bypass, reverse Trendelenburg is crucial to pull the colon and fatty omentum out of the way. Even routine cases such as appendectomy benefit from simple positioning changes: rolling the patient to the left and placing him or her in slight Trendelenburg elevates the cecum and allows the ileum to fall down and back from the field of view. In all of these cases, gravity is like a third hand retracting for the surgeon, keeping other organs out of the field of view. This is always a better method than constantly trying to sweep the bowel or omentum away so one can see the operative field. This seems obvious, but gravity is routinely neglected by the novice.

However, Restrain Gravity

Do not forget to use gravity and to protect the patient *from* gravity. For example, a common position for operating on babies is to place them at the foot of the table, with legs frog-legged, and the monitor hanging above the patient's head or chest. This position is excellent for Nissen, Ladd, duodenal atresia repair, abdominal approach to Congenital diaphragmatic hernia, eventration, Morgagni hernia repair, or choledochal cyst excision. However, the same gravity that pulls the omentum and colon down and out of the way can pull the whole patient down as well. However, for a baby, a little slip is a long slide: even 1 to 2 cm of movement is enough to dislodge the endotracheal tube. To avoid this kind of problem, careful padding and taping are essential. In addition, the use of a small bump under the abdomen acts as a kind of skid-stop to retard sliding (see **Fig. 1**; **Fig. 4**).

Add a Port

Adding a port in a case in which exposure or countertension is difficult can dramatically improve the overall precision and allow its completion more quickly. However, addition of a trocar seems to represent some sort of personal failing, a loss in a kind of *Name That Tune!* numerical contest in which the spleen can be taken out with 2, instead of 3 trocars. However, gamesmanship does not serve the patient.

An extra trocar will not contribute substantially to a patient's pain or scarring. If one is doing a laparoscopic procedure on an infant with one 5 mm and two 3 mm, adding another 3 mm trocar does not raise the pain and scarring by 3/11 (27%). Instead, the extra trocar site adds trivially to the patient's pain. Meanwhile, if the operative time is shortened from 3 hours of struggle with grasping and regrasping the bowel, into a smooth 1-hour case, the patient is plainly well served.

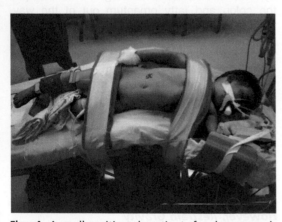

Fig. 4. A well-positioned patient for laparoscopic right nephrectomy. The surgeon stands opposite the kidney, facing the organ. Gravity is used to pull bowel away. However, gravity is also restrained. Observe that there is no stretch on the extremities that could produce nerve injuries, and that good padding protects from pressure injuries everywhere. No undercrossing lines or tubes snake beneath the body or limbs (these could quickly create pressure injuries in children). Note that tape with good tensile strength is used; relying on clear plastic or paper tape in an attempt to be gentle is a blunder; there is nothing gentle about falling off the operating table.

Consideration of trocar incision lengths brings up a prime fallacy about MIS. Inevitably, some critic argues that an operation that can be done through a linear incision whose length is similar to the sum of all trocar site incisions is just the same. For example, it is argued that a 2.5 cm incision is no different than five 5 mm incisions. However, it is not true that the lengths of trocar incisions add up to similar open incision lengths in terms of pain, scar, or disability. For example, it is intuitively obvious that 5 incisions distributed around the abdomen have a very low risk of dehiscence, but a 2.5 to 3 cm linear incision is vulnerable to this complication.

Incisional morbidity is a function of tension. Pain, scarring, infections, and herniation risk increase with increasing tension.[18] The mathematics of wound tension show that the total tension across an incision varies as a function of the square of its length not directly with length. Therefore, the total tension of a long incision is far greater than the summed tensions across several very small incisions of the same aggregate length (**Fig. 5**).[19] It follows that adding another small port does not contribute the same morbidity as lengthening an open incision. These smaller tensions across trocar incisions underlie the minimally invasive idea, but there is no reason for the surgeon to endure a minimal access disadvantage.

Do not struggle. Add a port.

MOVE WELL
Operate with Two Hands

When learning a new task, the natural tendency is to focus on the dominant hand, neglecting the nondominant hand. If the task is very new and very difficult, this unilateral neglect seems to approach that of stroke patients. Even the dexterity of the dominant hand suffers.[20] Unilateral neglect is nearly universal when residents attempt laparoscopy for the first time (a phenomenon not confined to laparoscopic surgery; every intern tends to ignore her or his nondominant hand when learning to sew). Novice operators struggle to manipulate a needle or cautery one-handedly, when they could easily help themselves with their nondominant hand. Instead, the instrument held in the nondominant hand drifts out of view, gets lost, tears the liver, or rips bowel.

The skillful operator moves both instruments in sync. Just as the 2 lines of music in a piano score merge into 1 stream of music at the keyboard, the 2 hands should always work together to manipulate the tissue. The tips of the instruments remain in view of the camera, and each move is slow, smooth, and controlled.

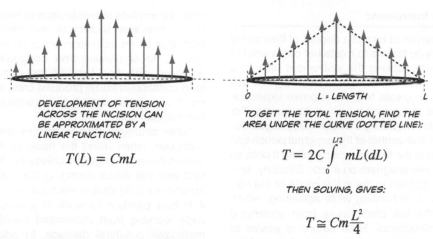

DEVELOPMENT OF TENSION ACROSS THE INCISION CAN BE APPROXIMATED BY A LINEAR FUNCTION:

$$T(L) = CmL$$

TO GET THE TOTAL TENSION, FIND THE AREA UNDER THE CURVE (DOTTED LINE):

$$T = 2C \int_0^{L/2} mL\,(dL)$$

THEN SOLVING, GIVES:

$$T \cong Cm\frac{L^2}{4}$$

Fig. 5. Incisions to not simply sum. Tension depends not on the length, but on the square of the length. It follows that adding a small port is minimally morbid, that smaller ports are preferred, and that single-port methods have a disadvantage.

Good teachers stress nondominant hand awareness with the refrain, "What is the other hand doing now?" Repeatedly redirecting attention to both hands allows the trainee to use both hands effectively and automatically. As musicians and athletes have long known, this kind of focused, immediate, specific, try-it-now kind of feedback defines the effective coach anywhere, including the operating room.[21]

Humans gain precision in fine-motor tasks when both hands appear in the visual field, even if one hand is not participating in the action.[22] To verify this, try cutting suture with one hand on one's chest versus with both hands in the field. With both hands in view, the cutting hand will be smoother and more precise. The same effect holds in MIS. Precision MIS is always a two-handed proposition.

Always Teach Two-Handed Operating

This leads to a common, but ill-advised, training method. Often, the attending surgeon arranges the case so that he or she manipulates organs with one instrument, whereas the trainee tries to operate with one hand and drive the camera with the other. Perhaps senior surgeons tire of camera work. Perhaps they feel nervous about the dexterity of the trainee and feel a need to have a hand in the action for control of the case. Perhaps they may worry that the trainee lacks the skill to use both hands. This practice always puts the trainee at a dangerous disadvantage. Attention is divided between 2 very different tasks, camera work, and fine dissection. Not only can these 2 tasks not be reconciled cognitively, but removing the nondominant hand from view degrades the coordination of the operating hand. Meanwhile, attempted

coordination between teacher and student resembles fencing more than operating.

Instead, the teacher is always better having the learner operate with two hands starting with their very first case, just as in open cases. If the teacher feels he or she needs more control, a solution is to add a port and an instrument, not to take one away from the learning operator. Another is to send the trainee to the trainer box with a coach. No one can learn to operate with two hands by doing cases with one hand.

Do Not Get in One's Own Way

Almost all novices seem to get in their own way. That is, they have a habit of grabbing tissue directly where the needle or energy tip need to go. Instead of controlling the tissue, they end up blocking the dominant hand or inviting other problems such as direct-coupling burns. It is often better to retract somewhat removed from the point one wants to cut or sew, creating indirect tension, or even to push down on some adjacent structure, thereby pushing the object of focus up into view. Operating with two hands means that the hands do not conflict.

It Is Okay To Be Ambidextrous

The skilled endoscopic surgeon is ambidextrous. There will be times when it is better to have the energy source enter from a left-hand port, and a retractor from the right. One should be able to readily switch instruments from hand to hand, always keeping the highest possible mechanical advantage. Trainees commonly shy from these switches, even if they sense the advantage. That is senseless; encourage them to try it.

Rotate the Instrument

A subtle example of loss of a degree of freedom is when a surgeon forgets to rotate her or his wrist or the instrument, locking the instrument tip into a disadvantageous position. In contrast, good use of rotation can create tension, improve exposure, or allow fine movement in very tight spaces. For example, when repairing a tracheoesophageal fistula, tension and control of the proximal pouch can be improved in the fixed space by rolling it onto an instrument, like spaghetti on a fork. Similarly, tension can be applied to the active blade of the harmonic scalpel by twisting while activating, which also pulls the hot blade away from underlying vulnerable structures. Even suture is easier to pick up after taking a moment to spin the tip of an instrument.

Use Energy Sparingly

Energy sources (electrosurgery, ultrasonic cutters, bipolar) create different tissue effects: cutting, coagulation, and coaptation. The effect produced depends not only on elevating tissue temperature but on the rate at which the temperature reaches above 100°C. In electrosurgery, the equation describing (roughly) tissue temperature change is:

$$dT/dt \cong \frac{J^2}{c\rho h}$$

T, temperature; t, time; J, current density = electrical current/contact area; h, conductivity; c, specific heat capacity; ρ, tissue density.

The parameters that the surgeon can control include current density and time (eg, how long the Bovie is energized). With a very high current density (eg, a small nibble of tissue, or application of the needle tip on the Bovie pencil), tissue rapidly reaches 100°C, water in the cells instantly vaporizes, the cells explode, and the tissue divides. With low current density, the water is driven from tissue slowly, the tissue desiccates, and coagulates. Knowing this, the surgeon can control the electrical energy precisely, controlling the effect (division or coagulation) as desired. A surgeon who does not understand this treats the Bovie as a magic wand and is puzzled when, for example, a greedy bite of tissue turns to a hard cord but never divides, even as heat spreads and damages to adjacent structures.

In small patients, the surgeon should take small bites (high current density) and use short acviation times. All energy sources perform better if the operator avoids getting greedy. For example, taking large bites of tissue to divide, a practice that, by reducing current density, leads to excess char, incomplete hemostasis, and broad collateral burns. Precision technique also benefits from a light foot (short activation time) on the pedal (or button). Most division and coagulation can be achieved with fine taps of the pedal, whereas long continuous burns produce char, stuck instrument, unsure hemostasis, and a wide penumbra of thermal damage.[23]

Other strategies add to precise energy use. In particular, when using the hook cautery, energy should never be engaged unless the tip is in contact with the tissue (swinging the activated hook around like a lightsaber risks cautery injury). Also, it is bad practice to work in a hole; keeping a wide working front maximizes visualization and minimizes collateral damage. In addition, good tension is indispensible.

Put Tension Where Cutting, and Cut Where the Tension Is

Perhaps the most important role of the nondominant hand is creation of tension on whatever area is to be cut. If allowed to fall slack (as often happens when the novice forgets the nondominant hand), the tissue will merely contract and char when energy is applied. Meanwhile, novices often cannot see that, although they may be creating tension in some tissue, the focus of this tension is away from where they want to be cutting. The tissue will not separate, but heat will spread and damage nearby tissue even as the operator vainly applies more electricity. In small spaces, unintended tissue damage follows this poor technique.

Scrutiny of tension lines and unfettered use of the nondominant hand allows the operator to recognize where the tissue tension lies within the tissue plane. However, tension is a moving target. The nondominant hand must continually adjust to bring new tension to the working plane while attachments are cut and tension is released. In general, the principle is to put tension where cutting and cut where the tension is. This sounds obvious but is notoriously difficult to apply in practice without an explicit effort.

DO THE SAME OPERATION

Unfamiliar anatomy and deficits in skills like suturing may lead surgeons to an operation that is pretty close, nearly as good, or a fair approximation. Stitches are placed close enough, short-cut methods with gadgets are chosen, and dissections are fudged in ways that the same surgeon would never accept if the case were being done open. These cheats are the origin of the shady reputation MIS sometimes carries. Who could be surprised when outcomes are inferior, especially early in a surgeon's experience?

Do the same operation means perform an operation with at least as good a mechanical result as would be achieved with classic open technique. This does not mean that every step used in an open procedure should be replicated endoscopically. Instead, one is aiming at the same final mechanical product.

Use the Same Suture

To perform an anastomosis with a series of fine, interrupted, monofilament sutures, do the same anastomosis laparoscopically. Alternatively, if a braided 2-0 on a ski needle is never used for this anastomosis, it should not be used laparoscopically.

Do the Same Dissection

Do not skimp on exposure (or, conversely, overdissect) with a switch to minimally invasive methods. For example, if the surgeon carefully isolates and visualizes the splenic vessels and clearly visualizes the tail of the pancreas during splenectomy, she or he should do the same laparoscopically, instead of firing a stapler semiblindly across the splenic hilum. If the surgeon mobilizes the colon more to decrease tension during an open pull-through or to visualize the kidney, she or he should mobilize it precisely the same amount when performing the procedure laparoscopically.

Perform the Same Mechanical Repair

The proficient surgeon has made a cognitive commitment to achieving the very same mechanical product. The ureter must enter the bladder at the same angle whether reimplanted by open or MIS technique. The fundoplication must be the same loose, untwisted shape using either approach. If a stitch is placed in that serosal tear in an open case, the suture should also be put in laparoscopically. The idea is to perform at least as good an operation, in which good is defined by the mechanical objectives of distributed tension, perfect approximation, correct angles, exposed plains, and controlled vessels.

Do Not Dither

The opposite case, loss of sight of the mechanical objective, sometimes manifests as a subtle halt in progress during a procedure. The error is not failure to commit to an exact mechanical result; the error is not knowing what the next mechanical objective is. For example, if the resident does not know what the critical view is in laparoscopic cholecystectomy, he or she will not know how to get there. He or she does not know what to do, yet feels an unspoken pressure to move along in the case. So he or she produces a series of aimless or repetitive movements, gripping and regripping tissue pointlessly. Clumsy and futile pushing or sweeping moves go nowhere, and the trainee grunts and sweats. At best, the case comes to a halt; at worst serious damage is done to delicate tissues.

This problem is called dithering. The remedy first is to recognize it, to stop the action, then to correct the root. Pause and reorient the resident to the next mechanical objective. For example, the natural tendency for humans when first retracting is to retract up or away, as with the cecum in appendectomy. However, this tends to hide the appendix behind a wall of bowel and even pulls the small bowel up to block the appendix. A better strategy is to roll the cecum down and to the patient's spine; that is, toward the operator and toward the operating room floor. This opens the field and tends to push the appendix up into view while holding down the small bowel.

Blink

This kind of view, and countless others (the correct pull on the rectum during dissection for Hirschsprung disease, the view of the opposite pleura in thymectomy, the mucosal bulge of the mucosa in pyloromyotomy, and the floppy smooth relaxed contour of a proper Nissen) are examples of visual patterns recognized instantly by the expert. Cognitive scientists give this sudden and highly accurate snap recognition different names, like blink, gist, fuzzy trace, or recognition-primed decision making.[24] In all cases there is a physical state of some system that is obvious to an expert but opaque to the novice. One object of surgical training (the most damaged by work-hour restrictions[25]) is achievement of this expert ability to just see some state through long exposure to many patterns.[26] With this experience, the expert can instantly see how to move from the current state to the desired state. The surgeon who cannot see this dithers instead.

SUMMARY

Skill is talent guided by method. The proficient surgeon has trained herself or himself to spot mechanical advantages where they exist or to create them where they do not. Mechanical advantage transforms clumsy technique into precision pediatric MIS, offering an antidote to the accidental moves tolerated during clumsy MIS procedures. However, regarding these principles as rigid rules or exhaustive prescriptions misses the principle of principles: principles are to be used, not obeyed.

REFERENCES

1. Morgenstern L, McGrath MF, Carroll BJ, et al. Continuing hazards of the learning curve in laparoscopic cholecystectomy. Am Surg 1995;61:914–8.
2. Morgenstern L. Warning! Dangerous curve ahead: the learning curve. Surg Innov 2005;12:101–3.
3. Garriboli M, Bishay M, Kiely EM, et al. Recurrence rate of Morgagni diaphragmatic hernia following laparoscopic repair. Pediatr Surg Int 2013;29:185–9.
4. Rangel SJ, Henry MC, Brindle M, et al. Small evidence for small incisions: pediatric laparoscopy and the need for more rigorous evaluation of novel surgical therapies. J Pediatr Surg 2003;38:1429–33.
5. Koyle MA. Minimally invasive surgery in infants. Con. J Urol 2012;188:1664–5.
6. Groves LB, Ladd MR, Gallaher JR, et al. Comparing the cost and outcomes of laparoscopic versus open appendectomy for perforated appendicitis in children. Am Surg 2013;79:861–4.
7. Brownlee EM, MacKinlay GA, Lam JP. Is it possible for traditional laparoscopic surgery to leave invisible scars? J Laparoendosc Adv Surg Tech A 2013;23: 78–80.
8. Varela JE, Wilson SE, Nguyen NT. Laparoscopic surgery significantly reduces surgical-site infections compared with open surgery. Surg Endosc 2010; 24:270–6.
9. Malkan AD, Loh AH, Sandoval JA. Minimally invasive surgery in the management of abdominal tumors in children. J Pediatr Surg 2014;49(7):1171–6.
10. Apelt N, Featherstone N, Giuliani S. Laparoscopic treatment of intussusception in children: a systematic review. J Pediatr Surg 2013;48:1789–93.
11. Hall NJ, Eaton S, Seims A, et al. Risk of incomplete pyloromyotomy and mucosal perforation in open and laparoscopic pyloromyotomy. J Pediatr Surg 2014;49:1083–6.
12. Dawkins R. The selfish gene. Oxford (NY): Oxford University Press; 2006. p. 360, xxiii.
13. Urbach DR, Govindarajan A, Saskin R, et al. Introduction of surgical safety checklists in Ontario, Canada. N Engl J Med 2014;370:1029–38.
14. Norman DA. The design of everyday things. New York (NY): Basic Books; 2013. p. 347, xviii.
15. Singh T, Zatsiorsky VM, Latash ML. Prehension synergies during fatigue of a single digit: adaptations in control with referent configurations. Motor Control 2014;18(3):278–9.
16. Zehetner J, Kaltenbacher A, Wayand W, et al. Screen height as an ergonomic factor in laparoscopic surgery. Surg Endosc 2006;20:139–41.
17. ElKoura G, Singh K. Handrix: animating the human hand. Proceedings of the 2003 ACM SIGGRAPH/. 2003.
18. Burgess LP, Morin GV, Rand M, et al. Wound healing. Relationship of wound closing tension to scar width in rats. Arch Otolaryngol Head Neck Surg 1990;116:798–802.
19. Blinman T. Incisions do not simply sum. Surg Endosc 2010;24:1746–51.
20. Desrosiers J, Bourbonnais D, Bravo G, et al. Performance of the 'unaffected' upper extremity of elderly stroke patients. Stroke 1996;27:1564–70.
21. Ericsson KA. Deliberate practice and acquisition of expert performance: a general overview. Acad Emerg Med 2008;15:988–94.
22. Georgopoulos AP, Grillner S. Visuomotor coordination in reaching and locomotion. Science 1989;245: 1209–10.
23. Massarweh NN, Cosgriff N, Slakey DP. Electrosurgery: history, principles, and current and future uses. J Am Coll Surg 2006;202:520–30.
24. Hudson D. Neuroanatomical basis for recognition primed decision making. Stud Health Technol Inform 2013;183:107–10.
25. Ahmed N, Devitt KS, Keshet I, et al. A systematic review of the effects of resident duty hour restrictions in surgery: impact on resident wellness, training, and patient outcomes. Ann Surg 2014; 259:1041–53.
26. Klein GA. Sources of power: how people make decisions. Cambridge (MA): MIT Press; 1998. p. 330, xviii.

Index

Note: Page numbers of article titles are in **boldface** type.

urologic.theclinics.com

Moving?

Make sure your subscription moves with you!

To notify us of your new address, find your **Clinics Account Number** (located on your mailing label above your name), and contact customer service at:

Email: journalscustomerservice-usa@elsevier.com

800-654-2452 (subscribers in the U.S. & Canada)
314-447-8871 (subscribers outside of the U.S. & Canada)

Fax number: 314-447-8029

Elsevier Health Sciences Division
Subscription Customer Service
3251 Riverport Lane
Maryland Heights, MO 63043

*To ensure uninterrupted delivery of your subscription, please notify us at least 4 weeks in advance of move.